THE
HEALTH
DELUSION

THE
HEALTH
DELUSION

HOW TO ACHIEVE
EXCEPTIONAL
HEALTH IN THE
21st CENTURY

Glen Matten MSc and Aidan Goggins MSc

HAY HOUSE

Australia • Canada • Hong Kong • India
South Africa • United Kingdom • United States

First published and distributed in the United Kingdom by:
Hay House UK Ltd, 292B Kensal Rd, London W10 5BE. Tel.: (44) 20 8962 1230;
Fax: (44) 20 8962 1239. www.hayhouse.co.uk

Published and distributed in the United States of America by:
Hay House, Inc., PO Box 5100, Carlsbad, CA 92018-5100. Tel.: (1) 760 431 7695 or (800) 654 5126;
Fax: (1) 760 431 6948 or (800) 650 5115. www.hayhouse.com

Published and distributed in Australia by:
Hay House Australia Ltd, 18/36 Ralph St, Alexandria NSW 2015. Tel.: (61) 2 9669 4299;
Fax: (61) 2 9669 4144. www.hayhouse.com.au

Published and distributed in the Republic of South Africa by:
Hay House SA (Pty), Ltd, PO Box 990, Witkoppen 2068. Tel./Fax: (27) 11 467 8904.
www.hayhouse.co.za

Published and distributed in India by:
Hay House Publishers India, Muskaan Complex, Plot No.3, B-2, Vasant Kunj,
New Delhi – 110 070. Tel.: (91) 11 4176 1620; Fax: (91) 11 4176 1630. www.hayhouse.co.in

Distributed in Canada by:
Raincoast, 9050 Shaughnessy St, Vancouver, BC V6P 6E5.
Tel.: (1) 604 323 7100; Fax: (1) 604 323 2600

Text © Glen Matten and Aidan Goggins, 2012

The moral rights of the authors have been asserted.

ISBN 978-1-84850-686-2

Interior images: p.49 © Aidan Goggins; p.288(top) Ross Harvey Photography

Printed and bound in Great Britain by TJ International, Padstow, Cornwall.

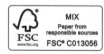

MIX
Paper from
responsible sources
FSC® C013056

To Olly and future generations to come.
Glen

To my parents, who didn't need years of
higher education to realize we need to
get back into balance.
Aidan

CONTENTS

FOREWORD

I first met Aidan Goggins and Glen Matten when they became students on the Nutritional Medicine MSc degree course that we run at the University of Surrey. We set up the course in 1998 because we perceived a great desire on the part of the public to know how to use nutrition to benefit health, yet recognized the fact that doctors receive virtually no training that equips them to give such advice. Since that time, we have taught many doctors and other health professionals how to use the peer-reviewed literature on nutrition and health to give a strong evidence base for their recommendations to patients and to those who want to optimize their own health and that of their families.

Aidan and Glen were both excellent students and wholeheartedly adopted our evidence-based approach, which has no time for anecdote or flaky science. Their desire to pass on to the public what they have learned, and to expose the fallacies and misconceptions that exist in nutrition and health, have spurred them on to write *The Health Delusion*. I wholeheartedly endorse their efforts and hope that this book will contribute to a fuller understanding of how nutritional information based on good science can be used to optimize health and reduce risk, both for this generation and the next.

Margaret P. Rayman, BSc, DPhil (Oxon), RPHNutr

Professor of Nutritional Medicine

University of Surrey

November 2011

INTRODUCTION

*'I believe that if you show people the problems and you
show them the solutions they will be moved to act.'*

BILL GATES, FOUNDER OF MICROSOFT, AUTHOR AND
PHILANTHROPIST (B. 1955)

The Health Delusion couldn't be more straightforward. It has one simple aim: to bring you better health. After all, good health is something that we've all come to expect in today's high-tech society, and who would argue with that? Unless, that is, we place this most valuable of things in the wrong hands. As we'll see, that's when it can all go badly awry. The end result is that the messages we receive are tainted and flawed and, rather than promoting our health, they end up detracting from it. So, before we rush headlong into helping you achieve our most simple of goals – the best possible health for you and your family – we've got to ask some pretty big questions. And that's where our story begins.

The first question we need to answer is, where has it all gone wrong? The advancements of the last century happened at breakneck speed, catapulting us into an age of breathtaking technology. The world we live in today would have been all but unimaginable just a few generations ago. Things once deemed impossible are now part and parcel of our everyday lives. The shackles that have held mankind back since time immemorial have been thrown off, and the possibilities of what we can now achieve appear limitless. We're not just talking about space travel or the cyber age, but medicine too. Health problems that were previously considered life threatening are now little more than minor irritants. Our lifespan is greater than it has ever been and continues to increase. When it comes to our health, we are fortunate indeed to live in this golden age of medical progress.

But there's a snag. Scratch away at this shiny veneer of health in the twenty-first century and what do we see? Sure, we're living longer, but can we honestly say that we're living healthier? Despite all the mind-bending advancements of modern medicine, a stark fact remains: if you are a healthy adult in today's society, you're in the minority. Does that really sound like the definition of a healthy society to you?

Don't just take our word for it – the statistics speak for themselves. More than one in three people has cardiovascular disease, one in six has high cholesterol and an incredible six in every ten has raised blood pressure. One in ten has diabetes and almost another four out of those ten are on the verge of getting it. If you see two women over 50, one of them is going to have an osteoporotic fracture. If all that isn't bad enough, two out of every five people will be diagnosed with cancer at some stage in their lives. These are devastating maladies that blight the quality of our lives and contribute to our premature demise. Does this unprecedented level of chronic illness and human suffering seem compatible with a high-tech golden age of medicine? We don't think so.

Let's get one thing clear: the crippling burden of chronic disease isn't a failure of modern medicine. Medicine has set out its stall, and that's to look after those who need it. It prevents the progression of disease and postpones death, and it's pretty good at it, too. To 'qualify' for medicine, we must first develop the ailments, the maladies, the symptoms and the risk factors. And this is where medicine belongs, as the last resort. As you'll see, all too often we place our faith in pharmaceutical drugs to solve our health problems, blissfully unaware of the true causes of ill health.

Worse still, we'll show you how the drug companies' attempts to medicate great swathes of society have mostly been an astounding failure. Instead of increasing our wellbeing, all they usually end up doing is leading us down a slippery slope of deteriorating health and drug dependence.

Here's the thing. It's this space, the bit between being healthy and the early development of disease, where the big problem lies. As for the answer, well, that can be found a little closer to home – in fact, for most, a little too close to home for comfort. Boil it down to basics and what we find is that our modern diet and lifestyle have become monumentally out of sync with what the body requires to stay fit, healthy and free of disease. Yet there's something that just doesn't stack up with all this, which brings us on to another of our big questions: how can our diet and lifestyle be to blame when we're so health obsessed?

With the mass of celebrity diets, health gurus, self-help books, glossy health magazines, wonder foods and supplements, surely we should be brimming with health? When it comes to conquering disease who needs more information than that to stay in tiptop health?

Yet, bizarrely, despite the endless procession of new-fangled diets, bestselling diet books and a thriving diet industry, we're more obese than ever before. What's that all about? And just in case you hadn't noticed, when it comes to obesity, things are rapidly getting a whole lot worse. Then we have a global supplement and 'antioxidant-added' food industry worth billions, not to mention the burgeoning array of so-called 'superfoods'. But have they put so much as a dent in the rising burden of chronic disease? Not in the slightest.

Sure, there are the common explanations, such as when it comes to health there's this great divide in the population. On one side there's the 'fast-food' generation, who are consuming nutritionally depleted and calorie-overloaded foods. On the other are those people who care about their health, munch down their 'superfoods', swallow their daily dose of vitamin pills and have the 'know-how' and discipline to diet, if they need to lose weight. We're not denying that socio-economic factors have a big part to play in health inequalities, but the problem is that the numbers just don't stack up. Right now, more than 50% of the population is taking at least one 'health' supplement daily[1,2]. That's before we start talking about the vitamins that the food industry adds to our everyday foods by the crateful. And the number of people who are overeating is actually far less than the numbers who are overweight.

None of this makes any sense at all, until you start to ask the big questions. As you'll see, we get some big answers that will make you think twice before buying another pot of vitamin pills or falling for the next celebrity-endorsed diet. So hang on in there, as we're about to expose the diet industry for what it really is: a fraud. Research shows that, rather than curtailing the obesity epidemic, it's fuelling it. As for the vitamins that so many people pop every day with due diligence, well, they could be promoting the very diseases people think they're being protected from.

But more of that soon enough. There's still another burning issue to tackle – the contagion of nutritional nonsense delivered to you courtesy of the media and self-proclaimed nutrition 'experts'. Even when we aspire to good health and are desperate for the answers, the reality is we often get fed bad advice. You can't open a magazine, read a newspaper, watch TV, or listen to the radio without being bombarded with health messages. It's just about mandatory that topping the bestseller book chart is the next great 'breakthrough' on how you can 'revolutionize' your health. At best, most of it is unhelpful, and at worst, it endangers your health. As we'll see, the media has a track record of misreporting the science, and most nutrition 'experts' fare little better. That we so often use this information as the basis for the important decisions we make about our health is, to us, scary stuff.

If the media and the nutrition gurus can't generally be trusted for advice, then where do we turn? If we want sensible, unbiased information, surely we can rely on our governments and health agencies to provide advice that is rational, scientific and based on the very latest research from the academic world. Well, we're sorry to say that's hardly the case. As you'll soon see, we have population-wide deficiencies of nutrients that are essential to our health and prevent many of the most prolific diseases of the modern world. But, not only are governments doing little to address this, they insist on clinging to their antiquated recommendations. By failing to act, they become part of the problem, too. Even when it comes to securing the health of future generations, we're being let down by policy-makers who shy away from giving the advice that you and your children deserve. In fact, even the enshrined 'well-balanced' diet is pretty bogus, and you'd think they'd at least be able to get that right. Yet it barely reflects the kind of diet that research now clearly shows we should be eating to foster long-term health and resistance to disease.

It's not hard to see that this is one big mess that desperately needs sorting out. As we delve deeper into the fallacies and delusions, you'll soon start to see how those bewildering health statistics we posed earlier have managed to come about. But we want to be clear about one thing: we're not just here to criticize and dwell on the negatives. Ours is a positive message that we want all to hear.

This brings us to where the idea for this book came from in the first place. In the field of health science, compelling research is published all the time. It's not always easy to interpret and can often be tricky to piece together and see the 'bigger picture'. But one thing hit us hard. So much of the really important stuff being uncovered by research simply gets lost in the 'black hole' of academia. We're talking about information that could really transform your health and make a big difference to whether you stay well or succumb to disease. It either gets buried or is 'lost in translation'. By that we mean, you do get to hear about it, but through the filter of the media, the self-proclaimed health gurus or the food and supplements industry, and the message is horribly distorted by the time it reaches you.

We think this is a travesty and more than anything else, this book sets out to take the compelling and exciting knowledge gleaned from academic research and share it with you in its unadulterated form. The truth is that so many of the answers to the modern-day epidemics of chronic disease are already within our grasp. What if you didn't have to wait for miracle medical breakthroughs to cure heart disease, cancer, diabetes and the rest, but could halt them in their tracks right now? What if taking action today would ensure good health for you and your family, and for generations to come? What if you had the blueprint for healthy living and truly preventive medicine? Wouldn't that be evidence that we are truly living in a golden age?

The information you need is right here at your fingertips. If you want good health, it's yours for the taking. And that is exactly what *The Health Delusion* is all about. A modern-day guide to true health, fit for the twenty-first century.

For a full listing of unabridged references and abstracts, as well as discussion and the latest up-to-date research on all the topics covered in the book, visit us at **www.thehealthdelusion.com**

CHAPTER 1
SCIENCE FICTION

*'Journalism: A profession whose business is to explain
to others what it personally does not understand.'*

LORD NORTHCLIFFE, NEWSPAPER AND PUBLISHING MAGNATE
(1865–1922)

OVERVIEW

- Whichever way we turn, we're bombarded with information about how to eat healthier diets and lead healthier lives.

- Much of our diet, nutrition and health information comes via the media and self-proclaimed nutrition experts, yet all too often their messages are flawed.

- We show you how to wise up to their ways by understanding some basics about how research is conducted and what it really tells us.

- Armed with this knowledge, you will be able to see beyond the headlines and extravagant claims and make more informed judgments about your health.

When it comes to our health, the media wields enormous influence over what we think. They tell us what's good, what's bad, what's right and wrong, what we should and shouldn't eat. When you think about it, that's quite some responsibility. It's certainly something we took pretty seriously as we were writing this book. But do you really think that a sense of philanthropic duty is the driving force behind most of the health 'news' stories that you read? Who are we kidding? It's all about sales, of course, and all too often that means the science plays second fiddle. Who wants boring old science getting in the way of a sensation-making headline?

When it comes to research – especially the parts we're interested in, namely food, diet and nutrients – there's a snag. The thing is, these matters are rarely, if ever, clear-cut. Let's say there are findings from some new research that suggest a component of our diet is good for our health. Now academics and scientists are generally a pretty cautious bunch – they respect the limitations of their work and don't stretch their conclusions beyond their actual findings. Not that you'll think this when you hear about it in the media. News headlines are in your face and hard hitting. Fluffy uncertainties just won't cut it. An attention-grabbing headline is mandatory; relevance to the research is optional. Throw in a few random quotes from experts – as the author Peter McWilliams stated, the problem with 'experts' is you can always find one 'who will say something hopelessly hopeless about anything' – and boom! You've got the formula for some seriously media-friendly scientific sex appeal, or as we prefer to call it, 'textual garbage'.

The reality is that a lot of the very good research into diet and health ends up lost in translation. Somewhere between its publication in a respected scientific journal and the moment it enters our brains via the media, the message gets a tweak here, a twist there and a dash of sensationalism thrown in for good measure, which leaves us floundering in a sea of half-truths and misinformation. Most of it should come with the warning: 'does nothing like it says in the print'. Don't get us wrong: we're not just talking about newspapers and magazines here, the problem runs much deeper. Even the so-called nutrition 'experts', the health gurus who sell books by the millions, are implicated. We're saturated in health misinformation.

Quite frankly, we're sick of this contagion of nutritional nonsense. So, before we launch headlong into the rest of the book, we want to take a step back and give you a rough guide to how research is actually conducted, what it all means and what to watch out for when the media deliver their less-than-perfect messages. Get your head around these next few pages and you'll probably be able to make more sense of nutritional research than most of our cherished health 'gurus'.

Rule #1: Humans are different from cells in a test tube

At the very basic level, researchers use *in-vitro* testing, in which they isolate cells or tissues of interest and study them outside a living organism in a kind of 'chemical soup'. This allows substances of interest (for example, a vitamin or a component of food) to be added to the soup to see what happens. So they might, for example, add vitamin C to some cancer cells and observe its effect. We're stating the obvious now when we say that what happens here is NOT the same as what happens inside human beings.

First, the substance is added directly to the cells, so they are often exposed to concentrations far higher than would normally be seen in the body. Second, humans are highly complex organisms, with intricately interwoven systems of almost infinite processes and reactions. What goes on within a few cells in a test tube or Petri dish is a far cry from what would happen in the body. This type of research is an important part of science, but scientists know its place in the pecking order – as an indispensable starting point of scientific research. It can give us valuable clues about how stuff works deep inside us, what we might call the mechanisms, before going on to be more rigorously tested in animals, and ultimately, humans. But that's all it is, a starting point.

Rule #2: Humans are different from animals

The next logical step usually involves animal testing. Studying the effects of a dietary component in a living organism, not just a bunch of cells, is a big step closer to what might happen in humans. Mice are often used, due to convenience, consistency, a short lifespan, fast reproduction rates and a closely shared genome and biology to humans. In fact, some pretty amazing stuff has been shown in mice. We can manipulate a hormone and extend life by as much as 30%[1]. We can increase muscle mass by 60% in two weeks[2]. And we have shown that certain mice can even regrow damaged tissues and organs[3, 4].

So, can we achieve all of that in humans? The answer is a big 'no' (unless you happen to believe the X-Men are real). Animal testing might be a move up from test tubes in the credibility ratings, but it's still a long stretch from what happens in humans. You'd be pretty foolish to make a lot of wild claims based on animal studies alone.

To prove that, all we need to do is take a look at pharmaceutical drugs. Vast sums of money (we're talking hundreds of millions) are spent trying to get a single drug to market. But the success rate is low. Of all the drugs that pass *in-vitro* and animal testing to make it into human testing, only 11% will prove to be safe and effective enough to hit the shelves[5]. For cancer drugs the rate of success is only 5%[5]. In 2003, the President of Research and Development at pharmaceutical giant Pfizer, John La Mattina, stated that 'only one in 25 early candidates survives to become a prescribed medicine'. You don't need to be a betting person to see these are seriously slim odds.

Strip it down and we can say that this sort of pre-clinical testing never, ever, constitutes evidence that a substance is safe and effective. These are research tools to try and find the best candidates to improve our health, which can then be rigorously tested for efficacy in humans. Alas, the media and our nutrition gurus don't appear to care too much for this. Taking research carried out in labs and extrapolating the results to humans sounds like a lot more fun. In fact, it's the very stuff of many a hard-hitting newspaper headline and bestselling health book.

To put all of this into context, let's take just one example of a classic media misinterpretation, and you'll see what we mean.

Rule #3: Treat headlines with scepticism

Haven't you heard? The humble curry is right up there in the oncology arsenal – a culinary delight capable of curing the big 'C'. At least that's what the papers have been telling us. 'The Spice Of Life! Curry Fights Cancer' decreed the *New York Daily News*. 'How curry can help keep cancer at bay' and 'Curry is a "cure for cancer"' reported the *Daily Mail* and *The Sun* in the UK. Could we be witnessing the medical breakthrough of the decade? Best we take a closer look at the actual science behind the headlines.

The spice turmeric, which gives some Indian dishes a distinctive yellow colour, contains relatively large quantities of curcumin, which has purported benefit in Alzheimer's disease, infections, liver disease, inflammatory conditions and cancer. Impressive stuff. But there's a hitch when it comes to curcumin. It has what is known as 'poor bioavailability'[6]. What that means is, even if you take large doses of curcumin, only tiny amounts of it get into your body, and what does get in is got rid of quickly. From a curry, the amount absorbed is so miniscule that it is not even detectable in the body. So what were those sensational headlines all about?

If you had the time to track down the academic papers being referred to, you would see it was all early stage research. Two of the articles were actually referring to *in-vitro* studies (basically, tipping some curcumin onto cancer cells in a dish and seeing what effect it had)[7, 8]. Suffice to say, this is hardly the same as what happens when you eat a curry. The other article referred to an animal study, where mice with breast cancer were given a diet containing curcumin[9].

Even allowing for the obvious differences between mice and humans, surely that was better evidence? The mice ate curcumin-containing food and absorbed enough for it to have a beneficial effect on their cancer. Sounds promising, until we see the mice had a diet that was 2% curcumin *by weight*. With the average person eating just over 2kg of food a day, 2% is a hefty 40g of curcumin. Then there's the issue that the curcumin content of the average curry/turmeric powder used in curry is a mere 2%[10]. Now, whoever's out there conjuring up a curry containing 2kg of curry powder, please don't invite us over for dinner anytime soon.

This isn't a criticism of the science. Curcumin is a highly bio-active plant compound that could possibly be formulated into an effective medical treatment one day. This is exactly why these initial stages of research are being conducted. But take this basic stage science and start translating it into public health advice and you can easily come up with some far-fetched conclusions.

Let us proffer our own equally absurd headline: 'Curry is a Cause of Cancer'. Abiding by the same rules of reporting used by the media, we've taken the same type of *in-vitro* and animal-testing evidence and conjured up a completely different headline. We can do this because some studies of curcumin have found that it actually causes damage to our DNA, and in so doing could potentially induce cancer[11]. As well as this, concerns about diarrhoea, anaemia and interactions with drug-metabolizing enzymes have also been raised. You see how easy it is to pick the bits you want in order to make your headline?

Unfortunately, the problem is much bigger than just curcumin. It could just as easily be resveratrol from red wine, omega-3 from flaxseeds, or any number of other components of foods you care to mention that make headline news. It's rare to pick up a newspaper or nutrition book without seeing some new 'superfood' or nutritional supplement being promoted on the basis of less than rigorous evidence. The net result of this shambles is that the real science gets sucked into the media vortex and spat out in a mishmash of dumbed-down soundbites, while the nutritional messages we really should be taking more seriously get lost in a kaleidoscope of pseudoscientific claptrap, peddled by a media with about as much authority to advise on health as the owner of the local pâtisserie.

Rule #4: Know the difference between association and causation

If nothing else, we hope we have shown that jumping to conclusions based on laboratory experiments is unscientific, and probably won't benefit your long-term health. To acquire proof, we need to carry out research that involves actual humans, and this is where one of the greatest crimes against scientific research is committed in the name of a good story, or to sell a product.

A lot of nutritional research comes in the form of epidemiological studies. These involve looking at populations of people and observing how much disease they get and seeing if it can be linked to a risk factor (for example, smoking) or some protective factor (for example, eating fruit and veggies). And one of the most spectacular ways to manipulate the scientific literature is to blur the boundary between 'association' and 'causation'. This might all sound very academic, but it's actually pretty simple.

Confusing association with causation means you can easily arrive at the wrong conclusion. For example, a far higher percentage of visually impaired people have Labradors compared to the rest of the population, so you might jump to the conclusion that Labradors cause sight problems. Of course we know better, that if you are visually impaired then you will probably have a Labrador as a guide dog. To think otherwise is ridiculous. But apply the same scenario to the complex human body and it is not always so transparent. Consequently, much of the debate about diet and nutrition is of the 'chicken versus egg' variety. Is a low or high amount of a nutrient a cause of a disease, a consequence of the disease, or simply irrelevant?

To try and limit this confusion, researchers often use what's known as a cohort study. Say you're interested in studying the effects of diet on cancer risk. You'd begin by taking a large population that are free of the disease at the outset and collect detailed data on their diet. You'd then follow this population over time, let's say ten years, and see how many people were diagnosed with cancer during this period. You could then start to analyse the relationship between people's diet and their risk of cancer, and ask a whole lot of interesting questions. Did people who ate a lot of fruit and veggies have less cancer? Did eating a lot of red meat increase cancer? What effect did drinking alcohol have on cancer risk? And so on. The European Prospective Investigation into Cancer and Nutrition (EPIC), which we refer to often in this book, is an example of a powerfully designed cohort study, involving more than half a million people in ten countries. These studies are a gold mine of useful information because they help us piece together dietary factors that could influence our risk of disease.

But, however big and impressive these studies are, they're still observational. As such they can only show us associations, they cannot prove causality. So if we're not careful about the way we interpret this kind of research, we run the risk of drawing some whacky conclusions, just like we did with the Labradors.

Let's get back to some more news headlines, like this one we spotted: 'Every hour per day watching TV increases risk of heart disease death by a fifth'. When it comes to observational studies, you have to ask whether the association makes sense. Does it have 'biological plausibility'? Are there harmful rays coming from the TV that damage our arteries or is it that the more time we spend on the couch watching TV, the less time we spend being active and improving our heart health. The latter is true, of course, and there's an 'association' between TV watching and heart disease, not 'causation'.

So even with cohorts, the champions of the epidemiological studies, we can't prove causation, and that's all down to what's called 'confounding'. This means there could be another variable at play that causes the disease being studied, at the same time as being associated with the risk factor being investigated. In our example, it's the lack of physical activity that increases heart disease and is also linked to watching more TV. This issue of confounding variables is just about the biggest banana skin of the lot. Time and time again you'll find nutritional advice promoted on the basis of the findings of observational studies, as though this type of research gives us stone cold facts. It doesn't. Any scientist will tell you that. This type of research is extremely useful for generating hypotheses, but it can't prove them.

Rule #5: Be on the lookout for RCTs (randomized controlled trials)

An epidemiological study can only form a hypothesis, and when it offers up some encouraging findings, these then need to be tested in what's known as an intervention, or clinical, trial before we can talk about causality. Intervention trials aim to test the hypothesis by taking a population that are as similar to each other as possible, testing an intervention on a proportion of them over a period of time and observing how it influences your measured outcome.

The greatest onus is now on what's called randomized controlled trials (RCTs). These are the gold standard and the most rigorous tests for investigating a cause and effect. Here, the population being studied is randomly allocated to the exposure of interest (say a vitamin pill) or a placebo (a pill that looks the same, but has no active ingredient), the beauty being that they, and ideally the researchers, don't know who's getting what (a process known as 'blinding'). In essence, the only difference between the two groups should be whether they receive the intervention or not. When it comes to comparing the outcome between the groups, we can then be that much more confident that any effect from the treatment is a real one.

Ideally, all science would be backed by RCTs, in which case there would be much less confusion about what does and doesn't work. In the real world that just doesn't happen, though. RCTs are expensive, often impractical and limited by ethical considerations. Take cigarette smoking. See if you can find a RCT of smoking and lung cancer in human subjects. You won't because you just can't do it. How can you randomize and blind participants so they don't know if they are smoking or not? It's obviously unethical to do it too, as you can't knowingly expose people to smoking with the goal of giving them cancer. No one would conduct such a study. For these reasons, epidemiological, and in fact all the other types of research we've mentioned, are still very important and can provide an extremely convincing argument, as long as we know how to interpret them.

Not everything can be subjected to a RCT, but we take issue with the selective reporting of observational studies to 'prove' a point, ignoring RCTs that have been published on the same subject. As we'll see, this is a favourite tactic of many nutritionists and supplement companies, and sometimes this cherry picking of research puts your health in jeopardy. Don't fall for it.

THE SCIENCE BLAST

Although this book is based on the findings of hundreds of scientific papers, it's written so everyone can read and understand it. So in certain chapters where we felt the science stuff got a bit too technical, we separated it out and called it 'The Science Blast'. For those who want that extra detail, it's there for you to read. But if you don't, that's fine by us, and you can skip those sections without missing out on any of our take-home health messages.

THE PARTING SHOT

Media 'nutritionists' aren't a new thing and people have been bemoaning them for generations. Back in 1931, *The American Journal of Public Health* declared, 'We suffer in this country particularly from fads… because of the many statements of "food experts"'[12]. Almost a century later, nothing's changed. So if, like many people, you read newspapers, magazines and health books, we urge you to consider what you're being told, otherwise you could end up thinking all sorts of things that bear little resemblance to the actual truth. When it comes to the relationship between diet, nutrition, health and disease, it's pretty complicated, and that's probably why a lot of it gets misreported. While there are undoubtedly people misusing the science to push their own agenda and sell their products, a lot of it is just uncritical and naïve reporting. Either way, wise-up and don't put your health in their hands.

SUMMARY AND RECOMMENDATIONS

- When it comes to diet, nutrition and health, don't believe everything you read. Far too much reporting is partial and misleading, and it shouldn't form the basis for dramatic changes to your diet or lifestyle.
- Cell culture and animal studies simply provide background information and are usually of limited relevance to your health.
- Observational studies of large populations never provide conclusive evidence – even when they are biologically plausible we may be confident but never totally certain.
- More definitive proof of cause and effect is achieved by conducting Randomized Controlled Trials (RCTs), although this 'gold standard' of evidence is not always available.

PART I
ANTIOXIDANT ALLURE

'In the middle ages, people took potions for their ailments. In the 19th century they took snake oil. Citizens of today's shiny, technological age are too modern for that. They take antioxidants.'

CHARLES KRAUTHAMMER, PHYSICIAN AND
PULITZER PRIZE-WINNING COLUMNIST (B. 1950)

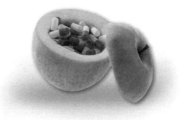

CHAPTER 2
FOOL'S GOLD

OVERVIEW

- Antioxidants have been one of THE big health buzzwords of recent decades.
- Bold health claims have spawned an industry worth billions.
- We expose how the hype for some of these 'health' products is founded on a flawed interpretation of the scientific evidence.
- We reveal why more is definitely not better when it comes to antioxidants, and why popping these pills may do you more harm than good.

Antioxidants. What a mighty word that has become. It resonates with health and holds the promise of great things. Antioxidants are enshrined in the language of the health-conscious and credited with quasi-mythical powers. An elixir so potent they can stop cancer, heart disease, and indeed the very ageing process itself, dead in their tracks. It seems the search is over, and the secret to eternal youth is ours at last.

CUT!

It might all sound decidedly familiar, but it's really a lot of old drivel. Nutritional propaganda fed to us by a food and supplements industry cashing in to the tune of billions. But it's not just the false promise of astounding health benefits that rankles with us. Sure, that's bad, but the fact that your antioxidant pills could be harming your health is what really gets us going, so we're out to derail the antioxidant bandwagon once and for all.

A modern-day panacea?

It was way back in the late 1950s that the American scientist Denham Harman proposed that the ageing process, and its related maladies, were a consequence of free-radical activity. On the surface, this makes good sense. Free radicals are unstable entities derived from oxygen that set in motion a cascade of damage to cells in the body, mercilessly targeting the likes of proteins, membranes and even our genetic material, DNA. As you might imagine, this trail of destruction is not without its consequences, which is why free radicals have been implicated in cardiovascular disease, neurodegenerative disease, autoimmune conditions and diabetes, among others.

Harman's proposal went one step further, showing that the addition of free-radical inhibitors (aka antioxidants) extended the lifespan of mice. Backing this up was mounting evidence from lab studies which showed that dietary antioxidants effectively snuffed out these injurious substances. The most tantalizing discovery was dangling right in front of our eyes. Was it possible that a host of age-related diseases could be stopped in their tracks?

Epidemiological studies then began to look at the effects of diets that contained high amounts of antioxidants (as would be found from eating plenty of fruit and vegetables). The findings showed that such diets were associated with reduced coronary heart disease[1], incidence of stroke[2] and cancer[3]. Of course, there are lots of reasons why fruit and vegetables are good for us, but these impressive health benefits were believed to be primarily attributable to the antioxidants they contain, which halt damaging free-radical processes[4–7].

The floodgates were open and in poured the epidemiological studies. Vitamin E became big news. Intake of this fat-soluble antioxidant was associated with over a third reduction in coronary heart disease in both men[8] and women[9]. It wasn't all coming from diet either. In these studies, the greatest benefit was typically attributable to taking a vitamin E supplement. In addition, a review of vitamin C trials found that high-dose supplementation (>700mg/day) was associated with a 25% reduced incidence of coronary heart disease[10]. Those with the highest levels of vitamin C in the blood had a 42% reduced occurrence of stroke[11]. It wasn't just heart disease either; the same was true for cancer. Epidemiological evidence was strong in showing the protective effect of high vitamin C intake against non-hormonal cancers[12], with beta carotene a strong contender too[13]. The studies were stacking up. The antioxidant age was upon us.

> **i** A common free-radical reaction is the conversion of iron into rust. To think a similar type of damage could be happening inside of us! It's no wonder that antioxidants have such mass appeal.

> **i** Antioxidant supplements were catapulted from the back shelves to fame practically overnight. This was primarily attributable to the frequent focus on life extension by the American TV icon Merv Griffin in the late 1970s and early 80s.

Antioxidant mania

The seeds had been sown, and green shoots appeared everywhere. The impossible was now made possible. We'd hit the mother lode, stumbled upon nothing other than the elixir of life itself, a veritable Aladdin's cave of untapped treasure. Free radicals quickly became public enemy number one and antioxidants our saviours. Free radicals were dubbed 'chemical assassins' and 'terrorists' (comparisons were as far-fetched as the 'atomic bomb'). But we were told not to fear, as antioxidants would deliver us from their tyranny. When it came to free radicals, there was only one way to go: a policy of zero tolerance.

There could be no doubt: more was better and the solution came in the form of an antioxidant vitamin pill. Sales increased exponentially. Spurred by a health-conscious and ageing population, nothing could hinder the growth of this market. This wasn't a health craze, it was a global mega-business, as the statistics prove. Over half the US population regularly take supplements and the vast majority of these contain some form of antioxidant, making a sizable chunk of a staggering $28 billion-a-year US supplements industry[14–16].

> **i** Americans alone consume around 50 billion vitamin and mineral tablets each year, so ensuring that accurate information is disseminated should be seen as a major public health issue.

Right here, right now, we're firmly in the grip of antioxidant mania. The word represents 'health' to the public, and an audible 'ca-ching' to the food industry. In a fortified/functional food industry worth more than $190 billion worldwide, 'antioxidant-added' and 'antioxidant-rich' foods contribute no small part[17] and this is only increasing. In the words of 'The Supermarket Guru', Phil Lempert: 'It's clear that regardless of whether or not people understand what "rich in antioxidants" means, it is certainly a logo or a stamp that says "Buy me! I'm going to help you live forever".' Hundreds of new 'antioxidant products' are hitting the shelves each year, as industry rivals grapple to get a piece of the pie. From cereals to jelly beans, chewing gum to drinks, it appears anything can be made healthy by adding some antioxidants into the mix.

Fool's gold

It's a pretty cool tale, don't you think? Antioxidants, defenders of our health, rushing to our rescue, but that's exactly what it is – a tale. Over-dramatized and misconstrued, this is the stuff of science fiction, not science fact. And here's the paradox. Despite being submerged in an antioxidant-saturated world, instead of curing our most prevalent diseases, their rates have actually been increasing.

There are two sides to every story, and you've only been told one of them. First, you can curb your hatred of those wretched free radicals; as you'll soon see, they're not quite the pantomime villains they've been branded. After all, it would be a cruel trick of Mother Nature if oxygen, the most critical substance for our survival, deserves the rap for our demise. It would be the ultimate irony if the most dangerous thing we do each day is breathe!

But first, we'll dig deeper. All those studies into diet and vitamin supplements that we mentioned earlier were genuine and exciting, but they were observational studies. As we know, when it comes to real evidence, intervention trials rule the roost, and with the buzz surrounding antioxidants, lots of these got underway.

As the results were published, the sheen rapidly began to fade from the antioxidant gloss. The intervention studies showed no positive effects from antioxidant supplementation, and a worrying trend of increased harmful effects emerged too. The omens weren't good. Cancer, heart disease and mortality, the very things antioxidants were supposed to protect us against were increased in those who supplemented their diet with them.

> **i** We refer to the term 'meta-analysis' throughout the book. This is when individual studies asking a similar question are grouped together to give an overall picture. As such, they can be a very powerful research tool.

THE SCIENCE BLAST:
ANTIOXIDANT SUPPLEMENTS

If you've been merrily knocking back antioxidants pills up until now, you might want to brace yourself, for this won't make pretty reading. It's time to delve a bit deeper into the research.

Whereas epidemiological studies had observed a correlation between higher levels of beta carotene and a reduced risk of lung cancer[13], giving 20mg of beta carotene as a supplement was found to increase lung cancer occurrence in smokers by 18% and their mortality by 8%[18]. No effect for vitamin C was found for cancer either[19]. In a study of US male physicians, 500mg per day of vitamin C produced no improvement in the occurrence of major cardiovascular events, myocardial infarction, stroke, or cardiovascular or total mortality[20]. In postmenopausal women with heart disease, rather than providing benefits, taking 400IU of vitamin E twice daily plus 500mg of vitamin C twice daily, almost trebled the risk of dying[21].

For vitamin E, the RCTs showed no benefit at all in taking vitamin E in cardiovascular disease[22] or cancer[19, 23, 24] – the very conditions it's widely touted to protect against. Worryingly, the most recent data from a large RCT in the USA showed that giving vitamin E supplements to healthy men actually increased prostate cancer incidence by 17%[25]. Indeed, a meta-analysis of 19 vitamin E supplementation intervention trials showed that, when daily doses went above 150IU per day (and you'll find much higher-dose supplements on the shelves of your local health store), mortality started increasing in a dose-dependent fashion[26].

A meta-analysis of 22 RCTs found that antioxidant supplements (vitamins A, C, E, beta carotene and selenium) had no preventive effect on cancer, regardless of cancer type, and in fact suggested an increased bladder cancer risk of 50%[27]. Another meta-analysis of 14 supplementation trials looked at vitamins A, C, E, beta carotene and selenium on gastrointestinal cancer occurrence and found no protective effect. Indeed a 6% increase in mortality rates was observed[28]. The only supplement to show potential protection against cancer was selenium, and there'll be more on that in Chapter 4.

In 2007, a review of 47 RCTs, totalling 181,000 subjects, found that antioxidants increased mortality by 5%. Beta carotene was found to increase risk by 7%, vitamin A by 16% and vitamin E by 4%, whereas vitamin C had no significant effect on mortality[29]. The irony is that antioxidant pills are still heralded as an anti-ageing miracle!

> **i** It is clear that it is no longer science but market forces that are driving the macabre antioxidant industry. We have to seriously question why mainstream nutritionists continue to advocate such practices.

> **i** The situation could be even worse. As scientists are more likely to publish positive findings than negative ones, it's very possible that there are more supplement trials showing the harmful effects of antioxidants which have never even been published[29].

Radical thinking

We're not really sure how to put it any other way: the antioxidant 'experiment' has been a monumental mess up. Something went wrong, very wrong. Swept off our feet by the lure of eternal youth, our gung-ho approach has failed miserably. The reason? Our total naïvety when it comes to understanding free radicals and antioxidants.

Listen up, because the chances are that, despite everything you may have heard about antioxidants, nobody will have told you that in small amounts free radicals are actually essential to our health. Since day one they've helped ensure our survival, as we've been moulded and sculpted into who we are today. Although they've been branded as the bad guys, free radicals perform a host of important functions in the body. For example, we need them for signalling systems involved in the regulation of such vital things as the life-and-death reactions of our cells to stresses[30]. They're needed by the immune system to fight off infection; without free radicals, we'd be unable to fend off invaders. While implicated in cancer formation, they are now also known to stop the growth and cause the death of cancerous cells[31].

Given all the evidence, the role of antioxidants is a whole lot more ambiguous than we've been led to believe. Free radicals most definitely can be the 'baddies', but only when the body's coping abilities are overwhelmed – a term known as 'oxidative stress'. When we think of free radicals, we might do well to think of the 'hormesis effect'. This is a neat idea that basically says a little of something that is normally bad for us actually does us good, but causes harm when we are exposed to it in higher amounts. A good example of this is stress. Too much stress is bad for you, but we need moderate short-term stresses to function and stay healthy.

> **i** It is wrong to think that antioxidants are 'good' and free radicals are 'bad'. It's a lot more complex than that and it makes no sense to try and interfere with nature by taking high doses of antioxidants.

What we're left with is a delicate balancing act. Both too many and too few free radicals spell trouble. And, really, is that so surprising? The human body is a supremely intricate and complex system, designed with elaborate mechanisms to ensure that free radicals are kept in check. This is achieved by a series of enzymes (glutathione peroxidases, catalase and superoxide dismutases), as well as antioxidants (albumin, urate, bilirubin, lipoic acid, glutathione and ubiquinol). We enhance these natural defences by consuming minerals in our diet (copper, zinc, manganese, iron and selenium), which are required for these antioxidant enzymes to function optimally, as well as getting antioxidants directly from food. The trouble is, we thought we could become masters of this dynamic, complex, finely tuned, self-regulating system, simply by consuming large doses of antioxidants in the form of a pill.

Ultimately, by taking high-dose antioxidant pills, we end up overwhelming our bodies and putting this fragile balance out of whack. For example, the US RDA of vitamin E is 22IU. It should be pretty apparent that it's non-physiological to be consuming 18 times this amount, which is what you'd ingest in a typical 400IU per day supplement (in fact, it's not unusual to see recommendations for double this amount – 800IU – 36 times the RDA!). The same goes for vitamin C. A diet rich in fruit and vegetables will provide about 200mg per day, yet supplementation doses of 1g (1,000mg) or more are often enthusiastically advocated. Indeed, the research now shows that while in lab tests high doses exert antioxidant effects, in the body, mega doses of the likes of vitamin C and E can actually have the opposite effect and act as 'pro-oxidants'. For anyone popping the pills, we think that's a bit alarming to say the least.

> **i** It's all about balance. In large amounts the free radical nitric oxide is linked with neurodegenerative diseases, epileptic seizures and increased states of inflammation. Yet small amounts are so beneficial for the heart that it is even used as a mainstream cardiovascular medicine.

> **i** Exercise dramatically increases free-radical production in the body. Far from being a bad thing, free radicals actually help the body to successfully adapt to exercise. Contrary to popular belief, taking antioxidant supplements reduces exercise capacity[32], and interferes with exercise's well-known benefits, such as improving insulin sensitivity and boosting our resistance to disease[33].

The whole is greater than the sum of its parts

A gross misunderstanding of the nature of free radicals is only one of the blunders. The second is the horribly simplistic notion that giving a massive dose of one or even a handful of isolated nutrients will satisfactorily meet the antioxidant needs of the body. It's not hard to see how consuming a balanced diet, rich in fruit and vegetables, will nourish us with a plethora of different vitamins, minerals and phytonutrients, all working in synergy to enhance our health. It is this nutritional cocktail, courtesy of Mother Nature, that confers the protection observed in consumers of a diet rich in fruit and vegetables. It's pretty obvious that this is the right way to go about getting your antioxidants. Gulping down mega-doses of isolated nutrients was never the way it was supposed to be.

First, an excessive intake of some nutrients can actually diminish the effects of others. A prime example of this is vitamin E. Vitamin E is actually found in eight different forms in the body (alpha, beta, gamma and delta tocopherols and four tocotrienols), but usually supplement companies will only include one, alpha tocopherol. Yet gamma tocopherol is the major form of vitamin E in the US diet[34]. It's required to quench the peroxynitrite free radical, and high levels are associated with a fivefold reduction in prostate cancer risk[35]. When we ingest high levels of just one type of vitamin E, however, we kick out the other types to make room for it[36]. So, while alpha tocopherol is associated with a reduced prostate cancer occurrence, this is only seen when gamma tocopherol levels are high[35]. In our opinion, taking a high dose of one nutrient without regard to the others is a bit like playing Russian roulette with your health.

This principle is borne out perfectly in a meta-analysis of prospective trials published in 2008, which found that while vitamin C was associated with lower coronary heart disease, this was only true of dietary vitamin C, not supplemental[37]. This suggests that it's the full range of nutrients found in vitamin C-rich foods which confer benefit. The same was found for pre-menopausal women with a family history of breast cancer. Compared with the lowest intake, those women with the highest intake of vitamin C from food had a 63% reduced risk of breast cancer, but this reduction did not exist in those taking vitamin C supplements[38]. However, this doesn't stop self-proclaimed 'experts' pushing high-dose vitamin C supplements like they are the best thing since the smallpox vaccine.

> **i** Don't confuse the message. High-dose antioxidant supplements are very different from the physiological levels of antioxidants found in fruit and vegetables. While antioxidant pills are a bad idea, eating up your fruit and veggies is definitely a good idea.

Evidence suggests that high-dose oral vitamin C supplementation is one of the biggest money rackets going. The body doesn't like to go above around 200–250mg daily (funnily enough, that is exactly what a typical diet rich in fruit and veggies provides) and protects itself against higher doses[39]. It achieves this by reducing the amount we absorb and increasing the amount we excrete. By consuming these supplements, you are literally peeing your money down the drain (although apparently it is an effective limescale remover, so maybe the plumbing industry will be next to cash in on the antioxidant act!). It's likely that this inbuilt safety mechanism is why vitamin C supplementation appears to confer the lowest risk on disease and mortality compared with other antioxidant vitamin supplements.

> **i** Gram doses of vitamin C are often advocated for preventing and treating the common cold. Considering we cannot even absorb these mega amounts, it's hardly surprising that the evidence doesn't support this practice.

Even in cases of known oxidative stress, it is not the case that any antioxidant will do. For example, it's well documented that smokers are one of the few groups that genuinely need extra vitamin C. They have lower absorption, lower vitamin C body pools and lower serum levels[40]. As a result of increased oxidative stress creating greater demands, smokers need about an extra 50% of vitamin C each day. Yet, if we decided to go with beta carotene instead, which has been shown to be associated with lower lung cancer in the general population, we find that doses higher than those found in the diet (normal intakes are 7–8mg per day) will exert a pro-oxidant effect and increase cancer risk in smokers[18].

THE PARTING SHOT

Taking antioxidant supplements simply doesn't work and this has been known for years. Yet millions of people are being misled into ritualistically ingesting these substances daily in the belief that they are enhancing their general health and wellbeing. The food and supplements industry relentlessly adds antioxidants to every conceivable product, while high-profile nutritionists, supposed 'experts' in the 'science' of nutrition, still zealously endorse the antioxidant agenda. Maybe it's a genuine lack of comprehension of the science, or a stubbornness to expunge former beliefs, or worse still, a blatant attempt to cash in while there's still money to be made. It no longer matters, but whatever it is, they're putting your health in jeopardy and it's high time it stopped.

The free-radical theory of ageing and disease was undoubtedly a clever one. Unfortunately, the science has been hijacked and misused. We're in no doubt that the antioxidant 'miracle' wins the accolade of the number one snake oil of the twentieth century. And that's exactly where this 'miracle' should be left behind – in the annals of history.

SUMMARY AND RECOMMENDATIONS

- When it comes to antioxidants, we've been led down the garden path with the idea of 'more is better' – it's simply not the case and routine use of high-dose antioxidant supplements is a bad idea.

- Antioxidants showed promise initially, but the simplistic idea that antioxidants are 'good' and free radicals are 'bad' is flawed.

- It's cruelly ironic that it is the most 'health conscious' people who end up consuming the most antioxidant supplements, unwittingly endangering their health in the process.

- If you eat a balanced diet rich in fruit and vegetables there is simply no need to consume extra antioxidants. Isolated pills will never replicate real food and taking non-physiological doses will ultimately spell trouble.

- The antioxidant bubble has burst and in the next two chapters we'll introduce you to some of the nutritional components that deliver real health benefits.

CHAPTER 3
PLANT PROTECTION

OVERVIEW

- Antioxidant vitamin pills are flawed, and so we must turn our attention to natural foods to get our fill of antioxidant nutrients.

- We explore the wonderful world of naturally occurring plant compounds, aka 'phytonutrients', which have health benefits extending far beyond a simple antioxidant effect.

- Public health messages urging us to eat our fruit and veggies are all very well, but that's merely the beginning. There's a lot more we need to know in order to stave off chronic disease.

So, we've knocked antioxidant vitamin pills off their perch and concluded that mega-doses of isolated nutrients cause more trouble than they're worth. That's not to say we don't think you should be getting antioxidants, just that they should come the way that nature intended, which is via food. This means that it is time to introduce you to the new and exciting world of 'phytonutrients'.

Phytonutrients are the components of plant foods that are being extensively researched for their ability to promote health and stave off disease. Unlike the high-dose vitamin pills, these are the naturally occurring compounds we've been exposed to through our diets for literally thousands of generations. Common sense should tell us that this has to be preferable to taking something synthesized, mass-produced and taken in the form of a pill.

Whether we're talking about heart disease or stroke, cancer or diabetes, obesity or osteoporosis, there's a mass of evidence testifying to the health benefits of having a diet rich in fruit and vegetables. We have campaigns galore to get us eating more of the stuff. The slogans of '5 A Day' in the UK or 'More Matters' in the USA have become key public health messages. And who can argue with that? After all, plant foods contain a whole lot of nutrients that are good for our health, such as vitamins, fibre, potassium and, of course, antioxidants. The idea, however, that the health benefits of plant foods is all down to their antioxidant content is a massive over-simplification of the facts. Sure, they're important but, as we'll find out, the effect of phytonutrients on our health is much more subtle and intricate.

One thing's for sure: if you want to take your diet to the next level, it's time to increase your intake of phytonutrients.

Technicolour diets

When it comes to the modern 'standard diet', many people are eating in the televisual equivalent of black and white. More precisely, we're talking about the atrociously monotonous diets of 'beige' foods that are all too prevalent. Based on the mass-produced fodder of white bread, white pasta, potato products, pastries, cookies, cakes and any number of battered and breadcrumbed convenience foods you care to mention, they all have one thing in common — they're beige and bad for you. These are the archetypal 'empty calorie' foods, the enemies of health because they are devoid of vitamins, minerals, fibre and, of course, our newfound friends, phytonutrients. What's desperately needed in such diets is the injection of some colour courtesy of fruit and vegetables. There's considerable interest in how the naturally occurring plant pigments in fruit and vegetables could be protectors of our health, so let's check out a few examples.

One such headline-hitter is lycopene, which is part of the carotenoid family and responsible for the deep-red complexion of tomatoes. The effects of lycopene/tomatoes were demonstrated in a meta-analysis that examined 21 observational studies[1]. It found that a high tomato intake lowered the risk of prostate cancer by 11%. What's most noteworthy is that the risk fell further, to 19%, in those who consumed high amounts of cooked tomato products. Because lycopene is tightly bound up in the cells of tomatoes, mechanical processing and cooking frees it up and increases the amount we can absorb. One study observed that men having two or more servings of tomato sauce a week had 23% lower prostate cancer incidence, compared with having less than one serving per month[2].

> **i** Lycopene is better absorbed from cooked or processed tomatoes. The presence of fat helps to increase the absorption of lycopene, too, so enjoy your tomato dishes with a drizzle of olive oil.

> **i** Tomatoes come in three colours: red, yellow and green. Only the red variety provides lycopene.

> **i** Along with tomatoes, watermelon and pink grapefruit also offer a handy source of lycopene.

While no large-scale RCTs exist, it is encouraging to note that a study of 32 patients with prostate cancer found that consuming tomato sauce-based pasta dishes (providing a bumper 30mg of lycopene per day) decreased levels of PSA, a marker of disease activity[3]. Prostate cancer isn't the end of the story either – lycopene has attracted the interest of researchers for a diverse range of benefits, including reducing the risk of cardiovascular disease[4], osteoporosis[5], and even protecting the skin from the damaging effects of the sun[6].

> **i** Lycopene is the secret weapon of the junk-food fiend. With its large amount of mechanically processed tomato paste, covered with high-fat cheese, pizza offers one of the most bioavailable sources of lycopene. Tomato ketchup is also up there as a top-notch source, while plain tomatoes in a salad come bottom in the rankings.

So, getting a good dollop of tomato-based products into your diet seems like a good health insurance policy, with lycopene seemingly the star of the show. But don't think this is all down to lycopene's 'antioxidant' credentials. While lycopene does have antioxidant properties, you only need to consider the fact that vitamin E is found in the prostate at a concentration 180 times that of lycopene to see that it's unlikely to be the mode of action for lycopene's purported anti-cancer activity[7]. And, especially, don't think it means that a lycopene supplement will confer these same purported benefits.

Attention has now turned to lycopene metabolites, termed 'lycopenoids', which may offer benefit[8]. It may be that other nutrients found in tomatoes are required for this metabolism to occur. Or perhaps we have it totally wrong and lycopene is simply a marker of another unknown nutrient, or combination of nutrients, which does the work. Whatever the reason, it teaches us the age-old lesson that we'd do well to avoid the isolated supplements and stick to the whole food package instead.

Hailing from the same family of carotenoids as lycopene are the yellow pigments lutein and zeaxanthin. Although sunny yellow, they're tucked away mainly in green leafy vegetables, but are also found in egg yolks. Being the only carotenoids that accumulate in the retina, they are thought to safeguard the eyes from damage by absorbing potentially harmful blue light and quenching excess free radicals. It is postulated, therefore, that these helpful plant pigments may be particularly effective in protecting against age-related macular degeneration (AMD) and cataracts. In a US study of adults aged between 55–80, those with the highest intakes of lutein and zeaxanthin had an impressive 57% lower risk of AMD[9]. A meta-analysis of such studies concluded that, while benefit was not seen in preventing early AMD, lutein and zeaxanthin intake was associated with significant protection against the development of the more serious late stages[10]. In a US study of male and female health professionals, those with a high intake of lutein and zeaxanthin had a circa 20% reduction in the rate of cataract formation[11, 12]. And even lutein and zeaxanthin supplements look like they have value, with RCTs now beginning to endorse benefit from supplementation[13, 14]. But with the likes of kale boasting a mighty 18mg/100g lutein and zeaxanthin content, and spinach 11mg/100g[15], going for the green leafy vegetables will meet your needs, as well as providing an array of other healthful nutrients besides.

> **i** Age-related macular degeneration (AMD) is the leading cause of vision loss among adults. More than ten million people in the USA, and up to 50 million worldwide, suffer with the condition[10].

Why stop there? Whether it is anthocyanins giving berries their red, blue or purple hues, or the betalains responsible for the deep red of beets, there's a veritable smorgasbord of colours to tuck into, which all boast their own unique health benefits.

The 'f' word

All in all, adding colour to your diet can go a long way to jazzing up its health credentials. But fruit and veggies are merely the beginning of our quest for a bumper crop of beneficial phytonutrients. This brings us nicely on to the 'f' word. Flavonoids represent a rather nifty group of plant compounds found in both fruit and veggies (especially onions, apples, berries and citrus fruits), but also abundant in foods and beverages we may not immediately consider conventionally 'healthy', such as green and black tea, red wine and cocoa. These clever compounds are speculated to possess a whole range of benefits to our health – acting as antioxidants, lowering blood pressure, inhibiting inflammation, inhibiting cancer cell growth, and even protecting the brain against neurodegeneration.

We must journey all the way to the San Blas Islands off the coast of Panama to get a better understanding of the health benefits of flavonoids. This is the indigenous home of the Kuna Indians, where high blood pressure is virtually non-existent and, in stark contrast to what we see in the developed world, very healthy blood pressure is maintained even into old age[16].

At the turn of the twenty-first century, US Professor Hollenberg and his co-workers unearthed the Kuna's secret and found that their major source of fluid was a beverage made from locally grown cocoa. The cocoa is fantastically rich in a specific type of flavonoid called flavanols, and the Kuna inhabiting the islands drink in the region of five cups or more of this flavanol-packed beverage daily, providing a staggering 900mg/day. When they migrate to Panama City, however, and consume the processed cocoa available from the local grocery stores (which is devoid of flavanols) instead, their immunity against high blood pressure is lost. Not only that, when Professor Hollenberg and his colleagues looked at the rates of heart disease, diabetes and cancer in the island-dwelling Kuna, they found them to have a remarkably lower risk of death from these diseases than mainland Panamanians. Could it be possible that a diet extraordinarily rich in flavonoids could be potent in protecting against the major diseases of the modern world?

> ℹ️ On a weight basis, dark chocolate is only exceeded by a few foods – such as buckwheat hulls, the cereal sorghum and cinnamon – for flavanol content[17].

Results from short-term intervention studies lend credence to the findings, showing that cocoa-containing foods and beverages rich in flavanols improve endothelial function, reduce blood pressure and improve insulin sensitivity – all good things when it comes to reducing cardiovascular disease risk[18–21]. There is also intriguing data from observational studies, such as a study of elderly men which found that those with the highest cocoa intake had lower blood pressure and almost half as many deaths over a 15-year period[22]. In another study, consuming chocolate twice or more per week was associated with a 66% reduced risk of cardiac mortality in those who had experienced a first heart attack[23].

When it comes to chocolate, flavanols are the 'Golden Tickets'. But in the words of Charlie Bucket, 'I'll bet those Golden Tickets make the chocolate taste terrible'. Well, 'terrible' may be harsh, but flavanols do have a bitter, acrid taste, and so manufacturers of chocolate are not keen on keeping too many of them present. Typically, the greater the cocoa percentage the higher the flavanol content, and usually it's the 50–80% cocoa content that has been shown in studies to confer benefits. But even that's all very wishy-washy. Just take a look at the results from the USDA analysis of ten cocoa powders. They found a massive range of 0.77–53mg/g (it's believed the content is 30mg/g in cocoas made by the Kuna Indians)[17].

Differences in cocoa beans alone can explain up to fourfold differences in flavanol content[24]. Furthermore, while processing steps such as roasting, fermenting and dutching may improve flavour, they contribute to a significant loss of flavanols from the final high cocoa-solids product. So as a guideline, when it comes to flavanol content cocoa powder is greater than dark chocolate, which is greater than milk chocolate, which is, in turn, greater than white chocolate. But ultimately, ingredient lists are pretty useless for predicting actual flavanol levels. In the words of Professor Hollenberg, 'What the world needs is a label on each package that describes the flavanol content of the chocolate'[25].

> **i** When buying cocoa products in the USA, avoid those labelled 'cocoa processed with alkali'. This process of alkalizing (dutching) massively diminishes the flavanoid content of the product[17].

Time for a brew

Cocoa flavanols are just one example of a bountiful group of compounds falling under the umbrella of flavonoids. Tea represents an equally tantalizing flavonoid-rich offering and we're sure we're not alone in enjoying a good cuppa. While many people are firmly wedded to a steaming cup of black tea, it seems we would do well to 'go green' and sample the toast of the Orient. The flavonoids primarily thought to give tea its health-boosting credentials are a group of compounds called the catechins. And while black tea contains about 3–10% catechins, green tea boasts a whopping 30–40% catechin content[26]

> **i** Tea is the most commonly consumed drink in the world after water. On average we sip our way through a whopping 40 litres of tea per person every year.

> **i** Lemon juice or honey is a good addition to your green tea. The vitamin C from the lemon and sucrose from the honey have been suggested to enhance the absorption of flavonoids and protect them from degradation in the stomach[27].

Folklore from Asia tells that green tea consumption began more than 4,700 years ago when the Chinese Emperor Shen Nung ('Divine Healer') produced a pleasant, refreshing beverage with green tea leaves by serendipity[28]. It was much later that the beverage developed its reputation for medicinal and healing prowess. While in the West we have a penchant for the black stuff, in Asia green tea has remained the brew of choice. This habitually high intake of green tea has been proffered to be one of the reasons for the 'Asian Paradox': despite an extremely high prevalence of cigarette smoking, Asia, and especially Japan, boasts some of the lowest rates of cardiovascular disease and lung cancer in the world[28].

In a Japanese study of 40,530 adults, those that enjoyed five cups or more of green tea daily had a 16% lower mortality rate than those consuming less than one cup per day, and an even more impressive 26% lower mortality rate when looking at just cardiovascular disease[29]. It was suggested that even one cup of green tea per day may bring benefit. When it comes to matters of the heart, the catechins are thought to exert cardio-protective effects through mechanisms such as inhibiting oxidation, reducing vascular inflammation and preventing blood clot formation[30]. Green tea also appears to have some cholesterol-lowering effects with a mechanism similar to a weaker version of statin drugs[30]. When the trials were put together it was found that high green tea consumption reduced the risk of coronary heart disease by 28%, with just a single cup a day associated with a 10% reduced risk[31]. Alas, no similarly beneficial effect was found in drinkers of black tea.

> **i** Decaffeinated green tea contains far lower catechin content, with levels of EGCG (epigallocatechin-3-gallate) approximately one-quarter of caffeinated versions. And bottled green tea is a no-no when it comes to improving health, as its catechin content is virtually non-existent compared to freshly brewed green tea[32].

While the Japanese study didn't find any effect of green tea on cancer mortality, there's no shortage of evidence from lab and animal studies to say otherwise, with lots of clever mechanisms explaining how components of green tea, most notably epigallocatechin-3-gallate (or EGCG), could fend off cancer[33]. While this means little on its own, it underpins promising results from the bulk of epidemiological studies. Recently conducted meta-analyses have suggested that green tea consumption may lower the risk of prostate cancer[34], stomach cancer[35], lung cancer[36] and breast cancer[37]. For breast cancer the greatest benefit may be to prevent recurrence of the disease, with three cups or more a day associated with a 27% reduction in recurrence rate[37]. Another study raised a provocative finding, with results suggesting that if you start drinking green tea before age 25 the development and presentation of any breast cancer that may have developed in early life will be delayed until later life (post-menopause)[38].

Overall, while there seems to be a trend towards benefit in cancer, it is somewhat inconsistent, likely due to different brands and methods of preparation resulting in considerable variation of the flavonoid content in what is considered a 'standard' cup of tea. When it comes to RCTs, they are few and small scale. There is definite promise, however, that warrants larger studies. For example, green tea extract has been shown to prevent the development of high-grade prostate intraepithelial neoplasia into full-out cancer. In 60 men with the condition (which is believed to be a precursor to prostate cancer), out of the 30 given 600mg of green tea catechins a day for a year only one prostate cancer case was diagnosed. In the placebo group nine cases out of 30 were diagnosed (a number that would be expected)[39]. In another study of 39 patients with high-risk oral pre-malignant lesions, benefit was seen in lesion outcome after 12 weeks with green tea extract[40].

> **i** While green tea has been associated with reduced oesophageal cancer, drinking it at boiling hot temperatures can actually increase your risk[41].

Just in case you haven't been paying close attention, you might be thinking that those few RCTs are an endorsement that you can cut out the palaver of drinking green tea and take a green tea extract in pill form instead. Listen up. When researchers at the US Department of Agriculture's Agricultural Research Service recently examined 20 commercially available green tea supplements, they found they contained high levels of degradation products, with some even containing unlabelled ingredients. The researchers stated that the level of quality control was unacceptable, and while some decent green tea supplements exist you can't tell simply by looking at the label[42]. So, rather than take a supplement, the key is to ensure that you're brewing up a high flavonoid-content tea. That means not just briefly dipping the teabag. Use hot water (above 70°C) and brew for a few minutes, or long enough to release the catechins, but not so long that the tea becomes bitter and unpalatable.

> **i** Flavonoids can bind non-heme iron and inhibit its absorption. One cup of tea with a meal can inhibit iron absorption by up to 90%[43]. This is especially of concern for vegetarians, making it advisable to avoid consuming tea at meal times, or at the same time as taking iron supplements. Adding a source of vitamin C to your tea or meal (such as lemon juice) can reduce this inhibitory effect[44, 45].

Flavonoids are a large family with many members and we need to be aware that it's not just our total flavonoid intake that is important, but consuming a wide variety of different types. Many in the food industry try to put the benefits of flavonoid-rich foods purely down to their antioxidant activity, and imply that you can compare the merits of different foods in this way. As we know by now, all the evidence suggests that this is hogwash, so we urge you to just ignore this type of ignorance.

What doesn't kill you makes you stronger

We get even further away from the simplified idea that it's all down to the antioxidants when we look at research on cruciferous vegetables. This is the family of vegetables that includes such notables as broccoli, cabbage, cauliflower, Brussels sprouts, rocket (arugula), watercress and radishes, among others. What makes these veggies special is their rich concentration of a unique group of phytonutrients called glucosinolates, more than 120 different types of which have been identified[46]. Unsurprisingly, they're pretty hot property when it comes to research into cancer prevention.

It's worth taking a look at how this all works. Initially, the glucosinolates are biologically inactive. It's only when the plant cells get damaged (for example by chewing them), that a specific enzyme, myrosinase, is released. This enzyme transforms the inactive glucosinolates into an active form called isothiocyanates, and these are credited with cancer-protective properties. Indeed, there's a whole bunch of epidemiological studies that associate consumption of cruciferous vegetables with benefits for a wide range of cancers, such as colon, prostate, breast, bladder, lung, kidney and ovarian[47–55]. There is much less in the way of human intervention studies, although the effects of a 12-month broccoli-rich diet on global gene expression patterns in the human prostate gland found favourable changes to signalling pathways associated with cancer and inflammation[56].

i Cooking inactivates the myrosinase enzyme, which reduces the amount of isothiocyanates you get from your cruciferous veggies – eating them raw or lightly steamed is best.

It's when we look at how all this works that things start to get really interesting. Out of the window go simplistic notions that vegetables are good for us because of their antioxidants. It's a lot more complex than that, with studies indicating that isothiocyanates can prevent the activation of carcinogens in the body and assist it in disarming them[46, 57]. And here's what we think is a fascinating idea. Maybe isothiocyanates are actually like weak toxins that stimulate the cells of the body to defend themselves and in so doing up-regulate their production of a range of protective enzymes[58]. Could it be that by inflicting stress on our cells, isothiocyanates elicit a cellular response that makes us more resistant to disease in the long run?

Likewise, when it comes to green tea, don't be fooled into thinking the purported cancer protective effects come simply from its antioxidant properties. That's certainly plausible, but it's likely to be a whole lot more complex than that. Green tea could also work in a more indirect way to stimulate the body's defence enzymes against cancer, or, intriguingly, it could be its pro-oxidant effects that may help inhibit cancer[59]. Now you can begin to see how the 'rich in antioxidant' marketing slogans are rather absurd.

THE PARTING SHOT

Irish lore states that if you find a leprechaun's pot of gold hidden at the end of the rainbow, the leprechaun will be indebted to grant your wish. There may be no leprechauns, or pots of gold for that matter, but if you make sure you get the rainbow when it comes to your intake of fruit and veggies, you'll be well on your way to being granted the wish for good health. We might not know exactly why phytonutrient-rich plant foods are good for us, but we can be pretty confident that they are. What's also certain is that the vast range of naturally occurring plant compounds we encounter in our diet interact with our biochemistry in intricate and complex ways. The notion that their health benefits can all be pinned down to them being high in antioxidants is a fallacy. Or for that matter, the crass idea that the benefits of such a plethora of nutrients – many of which remain a mystery to us – could be delivered via a pill that merely isolates one or two components.

What this means is that we shouldn't focus on one single 'superfood', or worse still, a single component of a food, as some sort of 'Holy Grail' for disease protection because it just doesn't work that way. The smart money is on spreading your bets and including a broad range of phytonutrient-dense foods in your diet. Above all, remember one thing: it's whole diets that really count and not isolated components.

SUMMARY AND RECOMMENDATIONS

- Ditch the 'beige' and put fruit and vegetables centre stage for a diet packed with colourful phytonutrients.
- Consume two to three tomato-based products/sauces per week for the prostate protector lycopene.
- Protect against age-related macular degeneration by eating dark green leafy vegetables such as kale and spinach.
- 'Chocolate heals a broken heart' and a few squares of dark chocolate with a high percentage of cocoa solids (70% or more), or cocoa powder, provide a delicious cardio-tonic.
- Take a leaf from the Orient and swap some of your cups of black tea for green to boost your cardiovascular and cancer defences.

- Make sure your flavonoid intake is diverse; especially rich sources include onions, apples, citrus fruits, berries, legumes, grains and red wine.

- It seems that cruciferous vegetables pack quite a punch when it comes to cancer protection, so aiming for three to five servings a week is a good bet for reducing cancer odds.

- Remember, it is the complex composition of plants that confers protection, so don't be fooled into thinking that a supplement will ever match, or that 'antioxidant activity' claims explain their benefits.

CHAPTER 4

SELENIUM: A MISSING PUZZLE PIECE

OVERVIEW

- Selenium, a trace mineral, was identified as being important to human health more than half a century ago but remains a little known nutrient.

- Indispensable for fertility, thyroid function, antioxidant defences, immune function and cancer prevention, selenium has a big role to play in maintaining good health.

- Selenium intake is tragically low in most European countries, leaving millions in a state of deficiency and susceptible to diseases such as cancer, and little is being done to improve the situation.

- When selenium does grab the headlines, recommended doses are normally too high and could give rise to unforeseen adverse effects.

- Discover how to get just the right amount of selenium to reap maximum health benefits, while minimizing any risks.

It's unlikely that you know a lot about selenium. And if you do it is likely that your knowledge comes courtesy of the self-styled health gurus who erroneously trumpet the use of high-dose selenium supplements. Either way, in this chapter you'll find out just what you need to know about selenium, and probably a tad more for good measure. This means you can do one simple thing every day that could make a big difference to your health.

Selenium, which borrows its name from 'Selene', the Greek goddess of the moon, is a trace mineral, which basically means we only need tiny amounts of it. What could be more straightforward? As ever, there's a catch. If you live in the UK (or much of Europe for that matter), the chances are you're missing out on selenium, and that spells bad news for your health, including your resistance to cancer. The flipside is that if you live in the USA, the chances are you're doing just fine when it comes to getting selenium from your food, unless you've been misled into taking an unnecessary high-dose selenium supplement, in which case you could be creating some problems of your own.

Where did all the selenium go?

As little as 30 years ago, folk in Europe were getting considerably more selenium than they do today[1]. At that time wheat was imported from North America, where it was grown in selenium-rich soil. Yet things changed, and Europeans switched to home-grown crops instead. However, the selenium-deficient European soils meant that the staple source of selenium was lost from the 'daily bread' and European selenium intake has not recovered since.

Average intakes of selenium in the UK scrape in at a rather pathetic 43mcg per day for women and 55mcg per day for men[2]. This is in complete contrast to the USA, where intakes are more than double this, with women averaging 92.6mcg per day and men 133.5mcg per day[2]. So, if you're living in the UK, it is likely that you're not getting enough selenium and as a result are putting your health at risk.

Little selenium and the big 'C'

Selenium has quite an impressive résumé. It's a feisty little nutrient capable of delivering antioxidant and anti-inflammatory effects, as well as activating thyroid hormones in the body. If you don't get enough selenium you run the risk of a compromised immune system, cognitive decline and greater overall mortality. That's before we mention its important role in male fertility and female reproduction, auto-immune conditions and combating viruses[3]. Yet its greatest claim to fame is undoubtedly its role in cancer prevention.

 Every year over 3.2 million Europeans are diagnosed with cancer and 1.7 million will die from cancer[4].

Before we get too deep into this, we're keen to set the record straight. If you do happen to read or hear something about selenium, chances are it'll be referred to as an 'antioxidant'. The way selenium works is a whole lot smarter than that. It does increase antioxidant activity in the body, but not through a direct antioxidant action (say, like vitamin C). What's clever about selenium is that it increases the body's inbuilt antioxidant defence mechanisms (a family of enzymes called glutathione peroxidases). So, by getting enough selenium in your diet, your body's 'nature-knows-best' antioxidant system can work to its full potential.

There are lots of very plausible ways in which selenium could help protect against cancer. First, selenium helps to reduce oxidative stress, damage to our DNA and inflammation, which are all implicated in the development of cancer[5]. Second, selenium can up-regulate the immune system, thereby helping the body to destroy cancer cells[6, 7]. And last, but by no means least, it appears that some metabolites of selenium, such as methyl selenol, may exert their own range of anti-cancer actions[8].

Initial published research created a great deal of excitement about selenium as an anti-cancer agent. Out of scores of prospective studies most showed that having a higher selenium level lowers the risk of common cancers such as lung, bladder, colorectal, liver, oesophageal, gastric-cardia, thyroid and, the most well publicized of all, prostate cancer[3]. The real headline-maker though was the much-acclaimed National Prevention of Cancer (NPC) Trial, conducted in the US. Here the effect of 200mcg per day of selenium was examined in 1,312 individuals. The results were startling. Those receiving the selenium supplements had a 25% lower rate of cancer incidence over the seven-year period examined[9]. There was strong suggestive evidence of a reduction in colorectal cancer incidence, but the true benefit was seen in prostate cancer prevention, with supplementation slashing its incidence in half[10].

While impressive, this trial was too small to conclude with 100% certainty that selenium is definitely giving these benefits. For that, larger, bolder and better-designed clinical trials are needed. And this is where we find a fly in the ointment. Exactly such a trial was carried out for selenium's promising effects on prostate cancer. Contrary to what was expected, the trial yielded disappointing results. SELECT was a large-scale randomized, double-blind, placebo-controlled trial of 35,533 men from across the USA, Canada, and Puerto Rico. Participants were randomly assigned to four groups, who received either selenium (200mcg/day), vitamin E (400IU/day), selenium plus vitamin E, or a placebo. In September 2008, after a period of five and a half years, the SELECT trial participants were advised to cease supplementing, as no positive effect at all on prostate cancer incidence had been observed[11]. Superficially at least, this seemed to blow the selenium–cancer hypothesis out of the water. But closer scrutiny tells a different story.

Not too much, not too little

What's going on here might sound a bit technical but it's actually pretty straightforward, so hang in there. What these studies tell us is that selenium demonstrates a U-shaped dose response relationship with cancer. This means that, as selenium levels increase, the risk of cancer decreases, but once you get to a certain point the risk plateaus, and if you continue to increase selenium levels yet further, the risk starts to increase again. For want of a better saying, when it comes to selenium, the old adage that 'everything is good in moderation' applies. What that means for you is that you should aim to get your selenium levels into the zone of maximum benefit – neither too low nor too high.

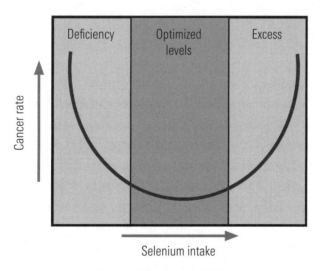

Selenium and cancer – a U-shaped curve

The way that selenium works is to do with the fact it's indispensable to a whole series of vital proteins called selenoproteins, which carry out a heap of good work in the body critical for everything from thyroid hormones and male fertility to anti-inflammatory and anti-cancer effects. There are 25 different selenoproteins in humans, of which selenoprotein P is considered particularly important when it comes to cancer prevention[8, 12]. Plasma selenium levels of around 120–125mcg/L (levels commonly seen in the US) are deemed to optimize the expression of selenoprotein P[12, 13] (the UK population languishes significantly below this threshold, at typically 80–90mcg/L[14]). Go above these levels and no further expression of selenoproteins takes place. It's almost as if you've reached saturation point.

> **i** In the words of Professor M. Rayman, Professor of Nutritional Medicine at the University of Surrey: 'Any condition associated with increased oxidative stress or inflammation might be expected to be influenced by selenium status. There is some evidence that this is the case in pre-eclampsia, pancreatitis, asthma, and systemic inflammatory response syndrome.'

What the evidence tells us is that the benefit from selenium supplementation is only realized in individuals that start off with low levels. Here we're talking about the kind of levels that are lower than we might typically see in the USA, but very common in Europe. The NPC trial, despite being carried out in the USA, was conducted in the southeastern part of the country, an area that has comparatively low selenium levels. Starting from this low baseline level, the trial found a significant benefit from selenium supplementation on cancer incidence. Yet this was not representative of the US population as a whole. SELECT's much greater population of 35,533 was a better representation. In SELECT, 78% of individuals had ideal selenium levels before commencing supplementation, which explains why no benefit was observed when they were given a selenium supplement. In fact, research is now finding that giving more selenium to people who already have sufficient levels is harmful for their health. Instead of preventing cancer it appears the risk may increase[9], and higher selenium intakes are also linked with an increased occurrence of diabetes[11, 15].

How much to take

As you can see, giving extra selenium to folk in the USA who already get enough is not the smartest idea, and supplementation is unwarranted. But for people living in Northern and Western Europe, who simply don't get enough selenium in the first place, it is recommended. Even so, doses as high as 200mcg, as used in the clinical trials, are completely unnecessary. We just need enough to match our US counterparts to optimize our selenoproteins. For women, a selenium supplement of 50–60mcg daily will raise levels into this ideal range. For men, especially those wishing to prevent prostate cancer, it may be prudent to go slightly higher, up to as much as 100mcg daily. When choosing a selenium supplement, we recommend that you take it in the form of selenium yeast, which best resembles food-form selenium and was the form used in the NPC trial.

> **i** Brazil nuts are touted as an exceptional source of selenium. We don't buy into that idea and suggest you don't either. Not only is the selenium content of Brazil nuts highly variable (more than a 1000-fold difference), they can also contain undesirably high levels of barium and radium, a radioactive material[3].

Where the message has gone wrong

While the early research made a case for the merits of high-dose supplementation, as we now know, more is definitely not better. To us, it's amazing that so called 'nutritionists' in the public eye, who were outspoken advocates of high-dose selenium supplementation, continue to remain part of the 'more must be better' brigade. High doses are indiscriminately recommended for European and US populations alike, despite ill-effects now being associated with such amounts.

Endorsement by American nutritionists of 200mcg supplements, the dose found to be at best useless and likely harmful, remains prevalent, and it's not difficult to find recommendations and supplements available for sale at outright dangerous levels of 400mcg. In the UK we've dropped the ball, too, by not understanding the 'U-shaped' concept. One renowned UK 'nutritionist' – who we won't name and shame as he is in no way alone – recommends 'a supplement of 200–300mcg of selenium for those who want optimal (cancer) protection'.

> **i** It's easy to envisage selenium as harmful in large amounts when we remember that it was first identified as a toxic element!

At the other extreme, and in many ways worse, is the lack of intervention from national health authorities across Europe. Some countries, such as Finland, have recognized their responsibility to the health of their citizens and ordered selenium to be added to the fertilizers used to grow crops, thereby bolstering intakes. The majority of deficient European countries, however, are yet to embrace such action (although ironically, in the UK we've been supplementing the feed of our livestock with selenium to reduce their disease incidence since 1978!). With more and more evidence demonstrating the benefits of getting adequate selenium, we have to seriously question why those with the power to act to boost our selenium intake are doing precious little about it.

THE PARTING SHOT

Above all else, we urge you to remember one thing: the 'U-shaped' curve. The USA and Europe are completely different with respect to their selenium levels. In the USA, a substantial proportion of the population already gets their fill of selenium, and vastly expensive trials designed to give even more selenium have consequently been a flop. Here the message is clear: if you're already getting enough selenium taking even more will have no benefits and could cause harm. If we've learned anything at all from the whole antioxidant debacle it's that over-zealous and excessive supplementation is a bad idea.

In contrast, it's the UK and Europe that urgently need the extra selenium, and right now they're not getting it. Here, to reap the benefits of this powerful trace mineral, a modest supplement is required. Even then, remember that the dose is key and it should be a selenium supplement designed to give the body just the amount of selenium it needs for optimal disease protection – no more, no less.

SUMMARY AND RECOMMENDATIONS

- An adequate intake of selenium, sufficient to optimize the functioning of selenoproteins, appears necessary for optimal health and to reduce cancer incidence.

- While most people living in the USA are already getting enough selenium in their diet, the UK languishes significantly behind.

- Good dietary sources of selenium include fish, shellfish, meat, kidneys and liver, but even eating a healthy and well-balanced diet is unlikely to provide optimal levels of selenium in countries such as the UK.

- For the average adult in the UK, a daily selenium supplement of 50–60mcg should optimize the functioning of selenoproteins and maximize anti-cancer benefits. For the prevention of prostate cancer, a higher dose of selenium, up to 100mcg daily, can be considered.

- Most people living in the USA are already getting enough selenium in their diet and don't need a selenium supplement.

- More is not better and excess selenium is outright toxic. Selenium is a double-edged sword, and having even marginally too much may have unforeseen adverse effects, including an increased risk of type 2 diabetes and cancer.

PART II
SUN SUPPLEMENT

'I think you might dispense with half your doctors if you would only consult Dr Sun more.'

HENRY WARD BEECHER,
SOCIAL REFORMER AND AUTHOR (1813–87)

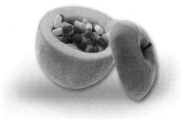

CHAPTER 5
'D'-FICIENT BONES

OVERVIEW

- Throughout our evolution we have been exposed to sunlight, which triggers the production of vitamin D in our bodies.

- Concerns about skin cancer mean that many of us avoid exposure to the sun, with the result that our vitamin D levels have plummeted.

- Vitamin D is essential for preventing the childhood bone disease rickets, but our vitamin D levels have become so low that we are now seeing a re-emergence of this virtually forgotten condition.

- This is just the tip of the iceberg: vitamin D is vital at every stage of life and we need it at far higher levels than are currently endorsed.

- We expose a developing osteoporosis time bomb, and a government with a lot to answer for when it comes to protecting our health.

At the turn of the twentieth century, the crippling disease rickets was prevalent in the industrialized world. With the subsequent discovery that a simple nutrient, vitamin D, could eradicate this scourge on children's health, you'd be forgiven for thinking that rickets was banished to the history books, and that the whole vitamin D story had reached a satisfactory conclusion. You'd be wrong on both counts. Research into vitamin D is red hot right now and the last decade has revealed some breathtaking findings. Some scientists researching vitamin D estimate that there could be as many as one billion people worldwide not getting enough of it[1], making vitamin D deficiency one of the most pressing medical conditions of our times.

Although it's the subject of some intense debate, when it comes to the health of our skeletons, only the most stubborn would disagree that we need a vitamin D level in the body of at least 20ng/ml for strong bones. Using this minimal figure as a guide means that a third of the US population is vitamin D deficient, increasing to almost three quarters of non-Hispanic blacks[2]. And, as we'll see in chapter 7, even these figures give a rather rose-tinted view of the true extent of the problem.

Cross the Atlantic and things are grimmer still. In the UK, during the winter and spring, over half the population have vitamin D levels below those needed for healthy bones[3]. Even in the summer and autumn, when vitamin D levels from sunshine reach their peak, significant numbers still languish below this threshold[3]. As improbable as it may seem in an era of high-tech medicine, there's even a re-emergence of rickets in the UK, particularly in ethnic minorities. So much for progress! Yet, as disturbing as the prospect of rickets is, more worrying still is the fact that low levels of vitamin D in the general population mean that our skeletal health is under serious threat, and the risk of osteoporosis and bone fractures looms large.

> **i** Vitamin D levels among the UK's South Asian population are of particular concern. Figures from Surrey, in the south-east, where vitamin D levels are typically higher than further north, show that 76% of South Asian women have levels less than 10ng/ml in spring, and even in summer the average level of vitamin D barely reaches 10ng/ml[4].

All this may sound alarming and depressing in equal measure, but the good news is that the problem is easily resolved by ensuring we get enough vitamin D. Simple. Well, we say simple, except for the fact that governments and health agencies are being monumentally slow when it comes to sorting out this mess. We're not prepared to wait, however, and will tell you how to safely boost your vitamin D levels into the range needed for healthy bones.

SCIENCE BLAST: VITAMIN D

All this fuss about vitamin D becomes a bit clearer when we look at its indispensable role in promoting a healthy skeleton. Bones need much more than just calcium. A bit like the great comedy double act Laurel and Hardy, bone health relies on the successful interchange between the duo of vitamin D and calcium. One of vitamin D's most vital roles is to increase the amount of calcium in the bloodstream. It does this by promoting the absorption of calcium from the gut, and also by acting on the kidneys to prevent it being flushed away in the urine. Getting more calcium into the bloodstream in this way encourages the mineralization of the skeleton. Vitamin D also has direct effects on the skeleton, helping to form the matrix of bone and aiding bone tissue to develop[5].

If vitamin D levels are low, however, our blood calcium levels are reduced and, in response, the body releases parathyroid hormone (PTH). This also works to increase our blood levels of calcium. Unlike vitamin D, however, it targets the body's greatest calcium stores, our bones. PTH triggers the process of demineralization, releasing calcium from the bones back into the bloodstream. To preserve the mineral content of bone, it is desirable to minimize bone breakdown by reducing PTH production by having sufficient vitamin D levels.

Vitamin D is converted by the kidneys into 1,25-dihydroxyvitamin D, or 1,25(OH)2D for short. This is the most active form of the vitamin, and at this stage it is more correctly classed as a hormone rather than a nutrient/vitamin.

Current UK recommendations are for vitamin D levels greater than 10ng/ml, to prevent the onset of rickets in children, and the adult equivalent, osteomalacia. But there is now a stack of evidence that conclusively shows that when it comes to vitamin D and our bones we shouldn't be drawing the line at this traditionally advocated cut-off

(10ng/ml). In fact, it's way off the mark. It should be two, or even three times higher (20–30ng/ml). Studies show that within this range calcium absorption[6] and parathyroid hormone suppression[7, 8] are maximized. If the fact that 15% of the UK population have levels below the absolute 'bare minimum' of 10ng/ml isn't shocking enough, when we apply the higher figure of 30ng/ml, we're looking at almost 90% of the population falling short during the winter months[3].

> **i** It is known that for every 10 degrees change in latitude away from the equator (where the sun is strongest) the probability of having a hip fracture increases[9].

> **i** In 2002, it was estimated that 44 million people over the age of 50 in the USA were at risk of fracture due to osteoporosis, or low bone mass. The economic burden of osteoporotic fractures in the USA alone was estimated at nearly $17 billion in 2005.

Stuck in the dark ages

The fact is that much of the current health advice is out of step with advances in the field of vitamin D research. Despite soaring rates of vitamin D insufficiency, the UK is the only country in Europe with no recommended vitamin D intake for 'healthy' adults. Even in vulnerable groups the recommendations remain a deplorable 400IU per day (an amount intended only to ensure levels of 10ng/ml are reached). Incredibly, the UK's National Osteoporosis Society, which is dedicated to 'improving the diagnosis, prevention and treatment of osteoporosis', released a unified statement with the British Association of Dermatologists, Cancer Research UK, Diabetes UK, the Multiple Sclerosis Society, the National Heart Forum and the Primary Care

Dermatology Society on 16 December 2010, stating that 'raising the definition of "deficiency" or "sufficiency" to higher levels (>10ng/ml) is inappropriate'.

We're just perplexed by this sort of advice. Just two weeks prior to this announcement, the highly respected Institute of Medicine in the USA published their recommendations after an extremely lengthy and thorough analysis, reviewing more than 1,000 publications. They affirmed that vitamin D has a pivotal role in skeletal health and that levels of 10ng/ml were simply too low. They determined that, for maximum benefits for bone health, the science backed a level of at least 20ng/ml (so, twice as much), thus making the UK recommendations appear even more out of touch. Earlier in 2010, Osteoporosis Canada increased their vitamin D recommendations to a minimum level of 30ng/ml. Furthermore, they recommended that all patients presenting with osteoporosis be investigated for the likely event of vitamin D deficiency.

> **i** While the UK still supports the antiquated view that a vitamin D level of 10ng/ml is sufficient, we urge you to ignore this recommendation. Instead, look further afield, to the USA and Canada, where improving the health of the population in this area appears to be a higher priority.

Storing up future problems

The whole situation is a mess, and you need only look at the state of bone health in the modern world to see why. One out of every two women and one in four men over 50 will have an osteoporosis-related fracture in their lifetime. In the USA alone, ten million people have osteoporosis and another 34 million have low bone mass, putting them at greater risk of osteoporosis in the future[10]. Put all of this in the context of an ageing population, and we have a recipe for disaster.

An old proverb tell us that 'prevention is better than cure', and to us, all these depressing numbers lead us to one inescapable conclusion: improving our vitamin D levels is not a luxury, but a necessity.

While we traditionally regard osteoporosis and suffering from fractures as diseases of advancing years, it's now apparent that promoting the health of our bones should be high on the agenda throughout our lives, in fact, right from day one. By developing strong bones in our formative years – what's known as achieving an optimal 'peak bone mass', usually attained by age 30 – the risk of osteoporosis in later life is greatly diminished. And getting enough vitamin D is critical every step of the way.

In fact, the importance of getting enough vitamin D for healthy bones begins before birth. It has been proposed that future risk of fracture might be 'programmed' during intrauterine life, with a mother's lack of vitamin D during pregnancy compromising how the bones of her offspring build up minerals early in life[11]. It's worrying enough that vitamin D deficiency is rife among mums-to-be, but if we add in the fact that a foetus is only exposed to 50–60% of its mother's circulating vitamin D levels[12], it's not difficult to see that we've got a big problem of vitamin D deficiency starting in-utero and in newborns.

But does any of this really matter in the long run? It appears the answer is a resounding 'yes'. In otherwise healthy pregnant women in the UK, having low levels of vitamin D during late pregnancy has been linked to reduced bone mineral content in their children almost a decade later[13]. Could addressing the vitamin D status of pregnant women be an effective strategy for stemming the rising tide of osteoporotic fractures in future generations? To us, it's obvious, but as we'll see in later chapters, it's still deemed perfectly appropriate to recommend an inadequate 400IU of vitamin D per day to pregnant and lactating women.

Let's jump on a stage. Vitamin D deficiency is common among children and adolescents, particularly during the winter months. In otherwise healthy US teenagers, the prevalence of vitamin D deficiency was found to be 42%[14]. In France, male adolescents had an average vitamin D level of a mere 8ng/ml, when measured at the end of winter[15], way short of what's needed for healthy bones. What impact could this have? Well, in post-pubertal girls aged up to 15 years, those with an average vitamin D level of 18ng/ml (which is still below ideal) had a 6.4% higher bone mineral content at the lumbar spine than those with levels of 8ng/ml[16, 17]. In young Danish men aged 20–29 (i.e. just hitting peak bone mass), those with vitamin D levels lower than 20ng/ml had a 2–3% lower bone mineral density compared to those with levels of 30ng/ml and above[18].

The consequences for the future of our bone health are worrying indeed. The reported changes in bone mass or density may not seem very large, but it only takes small changes to have a detrimental impact. Taking the last study as an example, if this seemingly small 2–3% reduction in bone mineral density was maintained into later life, this would translate into a predicted increased risk of vertebral fracture of 35%, and hip fracture of 80%[18]. Stack all this evidence up and we reach one conclusion: by not ensuring that pregnant women, infants, children, adolescents and young adults receive enough vitamin D, we're creating an osteoporosis time bomb.

Fractures and falls

It's high time that seniors got a look in too, as we ask the question: can vitamin D actually help to reduce the risk of getting fractures in later life? A large RCT in the UK found that raising vitamin D levels from 21ng/ml to 29ng/ml throughout a five-year period produced a 33% reduction in all major osteoporotic fractures combined[19]. A key finding from studies is how important it is to get your vitamin D levels above that all-important threshold of 20ng/ml, and the current UK recommendations for a vitamin D intake of 400IU per day just isn't enough. In a meta-analysis of 12 RCTs, supplementing 400IU or less had no effect on fracture incidence[20]. But in individuals who supplemented higher than this dose (averaging 482–770IU daily), non-vertebral fractures were reduced by 20% and hip fractures by 18%.

> **i** A 70-year-old has only about 25% of the capacity for making vitamin D compared to a 20-year-old. Couple this with a sedentary lifestyle and we can see that the elderly are a group at massive risk of severe vitamin D deficiency.

In the institutionalized elderly, supplementation with calcium (1.2g/day) and vitamin D (800IU/day) for 18 months reduced hip fractures by 43%, and the total number of non-vertebral fractures by 32% compared with those receiving a placebo[21]. Whereas measures of bone density decreased in the placebo group, supplementation actually caused an increase. While getting enough vitamin D is really important for preventing fractures in the elderly, it is worth remembering that vitamin D and calcium work in concert with one another, and optimal benefit is likely to be achieved from a combination of the two nutrients[22, 23].

> **i** The death rate within one year of suffering a hip fracture is between 20% and 35%[24].

There's a whole other dimension to the vitamin D and bone fracture story. As well as having a direct effect on the health of bones, studies have shown that vitamin D also improves muscle strength and function[25], which can significantly reduce the risk of falls. And once again, the key is to get those vitamin D levels above 20ng/ml. Compared with having higher levels of vitamin D (above 30ng/ml), having low levels (below 20ng/ml) is linked to worse physical performance and a greater deterioration in physical performance over a three-year period in both older men and women[26]. A meta-analysis of RCTs found that having a vitamin D level of 24ng/ml and above reduced the risk of falls by 23%[27]. Unsurprisingly, it was noted that vitamin D supplementation at traditionally recommended levels (200–600IU/day) had no impact when it came to reducing falls.

> **i** More than 90% of the annual 264,000 hip fractures in the USA occur after a fall, which means if falls could be prevented, it would greatly reduce the incidence of fracture[28].

THE PARTING SHOT

When all's said and done, there are two things that determine the risk of getting osteoporosis. First, the extent to which optimal peak bone mass can be achieved during the first two or three decades of life. Second, the rate at which bone is lost as we age. Getting sufficient vitamin D is vital for both.

This means we shouldn't just focus on older people in an attempt to reduce fractures (although that is clearly important, too), but need to start right from day one. Low levels of vitamin D are rife in people from all walks of life, at every age and stage. Traditional recommendations of 10ng/ml belong in the twentieth century. They should be at least twice, and maybe even three times higher.

SUMMARY AND RECOMMENDATIONS

- An adequate level of vitamin D is required for healthy bones at every stage of life.

- Traditionally, a vitamin D level of 10ng/ml has been seen as adequate, but current evidence shows this is not the case.

- For optimal bone health, you should be aiming for a minimum of 20ng/ml, and possibly up to 30ng/ml.

- Boosting your vitamin D to these optimal levels will help reduce the risk of suffering a fracture, and can significantly reduce the risk of falls.

- For maximum fracture prevention in the elderly, combining vitamin D with calcium is likely to be even more effective. Elderly people should aim to get up to 1,200mg of calcium per day through diet and/or supplements.

- In Chapter 7 you'll find out exactly how to boost your vitamin D levels into the most desirable range.

CHAPTER 6
'D'-FICIENT BODY

OVERVIEW

- Bone health is just the start of the vitamin D story. We unravel this nutrient's profound and far-reaching consequences for our health.

- Studies show that vitamin D influences our risk of virtually every modern-day health problem, including cancer, heart disease, diabetes and more.

- The breaking story is that the epidemic of vitamin D deficiency is leaving a vast burden of economic and health consequences trailing in its wake.

- Could vitamin D be one of the greatest medical breakthroughs of our times?

Nearly all the early research on vitamin D was dedicated to establishing its importance for bone health. There's a whole other side to this story, though, which has recently burst to the fore, with an explosion of research showing that vitamin D is crucial to many aspects of our health. We're not talking about a few minor health issues here, but some of THE most pressing health issues of our times. As a result, there's an almighty buzz about vitamin D.

Here's why. Low vitamin D levels are now associated with the risk of different cancers, diabetes, cardiovascular disease, multiple sclerosis, rheumatoid arthritis, osteoarthritis, pre-eclampsia, caesarean delivery, depression, Alzheimer's disease, infectious diseases and neurocognitive dysfunction. That's quite some list! Let's forget all the high-tech medical treatments for a minute: is it possible that a deficiency of a simple vitamin could be at the heart of our modern-day health problems?

It's a pretty mind-blowing thought, and one that's even captured the attention of the bureaucrats. During a parliamentary questions session of the EU Commission in 2010, it was announced that the 'economic burden attributed to insufficient vitamin D consumption is estimated at 187,000 million euros (260 billion dollars) per year'[1]. That's serious money. Disease, be gone. Financial crisis, be gone. Welcome to a vitamin D-driven utopia!

With all this going on, it's not hard to see why vitamin D is often described as the 'vitamin of the decade'. However, is this all too good to be true? After all, we all know how easy it is to get swept away with the fervour of something exciting, and before we know it we've lost all sense of perspective (just look at the whole antioxidants fiasco). So, without further ado, we're going to give you the real story.

Bring me sunshine

It all started with some intriguing observations during the 1930s, when a study of the highly sun-exposed US Navy found that their death rate from non-skin cancer was 60% less than in the civilian population[2]. Since then, it's been observed that simply living at higher latitudes (which means less sun exposure) is linked with increased risk of cancers such as colon, breast, prostate and several others[3]. Indeed, if you are diagnosed with breast, colon, prostate cancer or Hodgkin's lymphoma in summer or autumn (the times of year when vitamin D levels are at their highest), you have a much improved three-year survival rate than if you were diagnosed in winter or spring[4, 5].

We can draw the very same comparisons for cardiovascular disease too – a greater incidence occurs in populations living at higher latitudes, with greater increases found during the winter months[6]. And the list just grows from there. When it comes to a host of autoimmune diseases, such as Crohn's disease, type 1 diabetes, rheumatoid arthritis and multiple sclerosis, a similar trend between greater sun exposure and a reduced risk of these diseases has been documented[7–10]. With the discovery of vitamin D receptors on almost all tissues in the body, the sheer breadth and range of diseases that vitamin D deficiency has now been implicated in is simply stunning.

We could go on and on, so we decided to pin our focus on the big three – cancer, heart disease and diabetes.

> **i** Collectively, cardiovascular disease (including stroke), cancer and diabetes account for 1.4 million of the 2.4 million deaths in the USA each year[11]. Figures from 2004 show that these conditions were costing the economy an estimated $700 billion annually[12], and this has only increased since.

'D' and the big 'C'

When it comes to investigating the influence of sunlight exposure, the USA offers a unique case study. It's a country where UV exposure can vary considerably by region, even at the same latitudes. Of interest is the observation that there is a distinct east–west difference in cancer mortality rates across the USA, even though diets are broadly similar[13]. West of the Rocky Mountains, land elevations are higher and the stratospheric ozone layer is thinner, which allows greater UVB penetration and enhanced ability to synthesize vitamin D[13, 14]. Could something as simple as vitamin-D boosting sunshine explain the geographical variation in cancer mortality rates across the US? Let's see if we can get some answers.

A large US ecological study carried out between 1950 and 1969 and 1970 and 1994 found that those people living in areas with the greatest UVB exposure had significantly reduced levels of 15 different cancers[14]. This was true even after accounting for potential confounders, such as smoking, ethnicity, alcohol consumption, affluence and urban residence. So strong was the observed effect of higher levels of UVB exposure that the authors calculated it would equate to saving up to 60,000 lives each year – a staggering 10% of the US death toll due to cancer. (It's an interesting aside that in the 1980s the strength of this association decreased, corresponding with the introduction of anti-skin cancer campaigns to limit sun exposure, and the recommended use of sun block.)

As exciting as all this sounds, we should curb the enthusiasm just a bit by saying that these are all ecological studies, from which we shouldn't be jumping to any definitive conclusions. It begs the important question: how plausible is all this information? Could vitamin D really stop something as deadly as cancer in its tracks? If we look at what vitamin D actually does in the tissues of the body, then we begin to see how this could work.

We can think of vitamin D as being on sentry duty at checkpoints in a cell. If the cell is attacked (e.g. causing DNA damage), or if there's any reason that it's not functioning properly, vitamin D helps sound the alarm, as well as enabling cell defence mechanisms to kick in. Unwanted cell growth is halted and damaged cells are destroyed. Without this early guard duty, corrupted cells are allowed to grow and replicate in an uncontrolled manner. By the time our body's defences are alerted and mobilized, it's too late. They are quickly overwhelmed and cancer gains the upper hand.

Amazingly, there are more than 1,000 human genes with vitamin D response elements[15], with many involved in making important proteins that help to regulate essential functions such as cell proliferation, differentiation and apoptosis, all of which need to be tightly controlled to stave off cancer.

 Every two minutes, someone in the UK is diagnosed with cancer[16].

So far, evidence for a cancer-protective effect of vitamin D looks strongest for colorectal cancer and breast cancer. The National Health and Nutrition Examination Survey in the USA found that those with vitamin D levels greater than 32ng/ml had 72% fewer deaths from colorectal cancer compared to those with levels less than 20ng/ml[17]. This impressive effect was still seen even after accounting for BMI (body mass index) and physical activity levels – two factors which not only affect vitamin D levels, but also directly affect the risk of colorectal cancer. Rather than just being a one-off, these exciting findings have been borne out by other observational studies. In a meta-analysis of studies, which prospectively examined vitamin D levels in relation to colorectal cancer, having levels of 33ng/ml or more was associated with a 50% lower incidence of colorectal cancer compared with having levels of 12ng/ml or less[18].

When it comes to breast cancer, a meta-analysis of seven trials examining circulating vitamin D levels found that those with the highest levels had a 45% reduced occurrence of breast cancer compared to those with the lowest levels[19]. In a second meta-analysis of nine observational trials, raising vitamin D levels by 20ng/ml was associated with a 27% reduction in breast cancer occurrence[20].

In 2007, there were 345,636 cases of breast and colorectal cancer in the USA, with 93,817 people dying that year from these two diseases[21].

As we know, the evidence from observational studies is just a teaser, highly suggestive but never definitive. True evidence of cause and effect can only come from rigorously performed RCTs. Unfortunately, when it comes to vitamin D these are still very thin on the ground. In fact, there is not a single large-scale RCT of vitamin D where cancer has been pre-specified as the primary outcome of the study[22]. So, where RCTs do exist, we have to ask how relevant are they?

We'll take the Women's Health Initiative trial as our example. This found no effects of vitamin D after seven years on risk of colorectal cancer or breast cancer[23, 24]. But before you think this blows the whole vitamin D story out of the water, you have to realize that this study was designed in the early 1990s, before the big surge of interest in vitamin D as a cancer protective nutrient had gathered pace. The dosage used was a mere 400IU per day (and if you take the poor adherence of the participants into account, it would be much lower). This is virtually a meaningless amount and far below the higher levels that have been observed to have a protective effect against cancer.

The second RCT used a more meaningful vitamin D dose of 1,100IU per day. This raised the participant's vitamin D levels from an already very respectable 28ng/ml to an even higher level of 38ng/ml. This 10ng/ml rise in vitamin D levels was associated with a 35% reduction in total cancer risk[25]. Unfortunately, what seemed an extremely promising finding was tempered by considerable criticism of the study's methodology[26–28], including the fact that there were unexpectedly high rates of cancer in the placebo group, which may have artificially skewed the results in favour of vitamin D[28, 29].

So, we still need to await the results from more rigorous RCTs to truly prove the cancer link. But all in all, things look quite promising, and if there really is no smoke without fire, it looks like vitamin D is essential to ensure incineration of those malignant cells.

Cardiovascular 'D'-sease

Look up any list of cardiovascular disease risk factors and broadly speaking, they're always the same. You'll see the usual suspects, such as obesity, smoking, lack of exercise, elevated cholesterol, triglycerides and homocysteine, eating a lot of salt and so on. We're pretty sure that you won't see vitamin D listed anywhere. Yet evidence is mounting to demonstrate the necessity of sufficient vitamin D levels for heart health too.

> **i** While deaths from heart disease are falling, it still remains the Western world's biggest killer. More than 616,000 people die from heart disease in the USA each year[30]. Heart disease carries with it an annual economic cost of over $445 billion in the USA alone[31].

Results from the Health Professionals Follow-up Study support this idea. They showed that men deficient in vitamin D (<15ng/ml) had more than double the risk of a heart attack compared with men with higher vitamin D levels (>30ng/ml)[6]. In 1,739 participants from the Framingham Offspring Study, those with a vitamin D level less than 15ng/ml had 62% more cardiovascular events compared to those with a vitamin D level above 15ng/ml[32]. Another study indicated that the risk of being diagnosed with hypertension over a four-year period was more than three times greater in those with vitamin D levels below 15ng/ml, compared with those who had a level of 30ng/ml or above[33]. Having low levels of vitamin D has additionally been linked to increased risk of fatal strokes[34], heart failure and sudden cardiac death[35].

Vitamin D has quite some litany of benefits, but does it all stack up? How does it work its magic? Are these observations biologically plausible?

It appears so, as vitamin D works in a number of ways to protect the cardiovascular system – affecting the proliferation of smooth muscle cells, reducing inflammation, helping to control calcification of blood vessels, improving endothelial function, and even reducing blood pressure, all things that can affect the risk of heart disease[6, 36]

But once again, show us the well-designed RCTs? There's the Women's Health Initiative study again, but as with cancer, it's pretty useless and the lack of benefit observed was hardly surprising given the small dose of vitamin D and the low adherence of the participants actually taking the supplements. There have been a couple of studies which tentatively suggest that higher doses of vitamin D supplements (820IU[37] and 1,000IU[38] daily) reduce cardiovascular disease. But the results were not strong enough, nor the trials well enough designed to draw any firm conclusions, underlining the need for better studies to be conducted.

'D' for diabetes

As if protection against cancer and heart disease wasn't enough, evidence is growing that vitamin D may also prevent one of the other major diseases of our times, diabetes. It makes sense too, when you consider that vitamin D appears to be involved in the functioning of beta cells (the cells that make and release insulin), insulin sensitivity and levels of inflammation in the body, all of which influence how well we can handle glucose and, ultimately, the risk of type 2 diabetes[39].

> **i** Worldwide, the number of people with diabetes is expected to rise from 171 million in 2000 to a staggering 366 million by 2030[40].

> **i** Type 2 diabetes has serious long-term health consequences (it affects the kidneys, eyesight, gums, heart and nervous system), and simple ways of preventing it, such as getting enough vitamin D, are desperately needed.

In the USA, in 2006 alone, 65,700 diabetics had to have a lower limb amputated[41].

These fancy 'mechanisms' are all well and good, but what happens in the real world? A review of observational studies found that intakes of vitamin D greater than 500IU daily decreased type 2 diabetes risk by 13%, compared with vitamin D intakes of less than 200IU per day[42]. According to vitamin D status, those with the highest vitamin D levels (>25ng/ml) had a 43% lower risk of getting type 2 diabetes compared to those with the lowest levels (<14ng/ml)[42]. This is similar to another review, which found that having higher vitamin D levels (25–38ng/ml) was associated with a 64% reduction in the prevalence of type 2 diabetes, compared with those who had lower levels (10–23ng/ml)[43], although this link was only clearly demonstrated once data on non-Hispanic blacks was excluded from the analysis.

Concrete evidence from RCTs is required to establish proof. In just such a trial, diabetics were given vitamin D-fortified yoghurts providing 1,000IU per day for 12 weeks[44]. The baseline vitamin D levels at the start of the study were, on average, 18ng/ml, with 70% having levels less than 20ng/ml, and rose to an average of 30ng/ml with the intervention. The increase in vitamin D status corresponded to a significantly lower weight (2kg loss) and waist size (2.5cm / 1in / 2.5% reduction) compared to the placebo group, as well as improvements in measures of blood sugar control.

Vitamin D's anti-diabetes credentials are not just limited to type 2 diabetes, but extend to type 1 diabetes too. This is a very different condition, in which the body's immune system attacks and destroys the insulin-producing beta cells of the pancreas. In contrast to type 2 diabetes, which typically affects older people, type 1 diabetes is usually diagnosed in childhood. A low number of sunshine hours has been shown to correlate with the incidence of type 1 diabetes[45], as too has seasonal variations in diagnosis (higher in late autumn and winter, lower in summer)[8, 46]. Vitamin D levels have also been found to be lower in people at the time of diagnosis of type 1 diabetes compared with controls[47].

 Although type 1 and type 2 diabetes are very different diseases, vitamin D appears to help prevent both.

Vitamin D intake during pregnancy, lactation and infancy appears to reduce the risk of going on to develop type 1 diabetes. The immuno-modulatory effects of vitamin D are well documented and it is by these actions that the risk of type 1 diabetes is believed to be reduced. A recent meta-analysis concluded that supplementation with vitamin D in infancy was associated with a 29% reduced risk of type 1 diabetes[48]. In Finnish infants aged one year, the reduction in the incidence of type 1 diabetes in those who regularly received very high dose vitamin D supplementation was 88%[49]. Tellingly, in those infants suspected of having rickets, suggesting extreme vitamin D deficiency, there was a threefold increased risk of developing diabetes.

THE PARTING SHOT

It's now crystal clear that vitamin D plays a far more complex role in the body than simply being important for healthy bones. With the vitamin D receptor expressed in most tissues of the body, it's hardly surprising that a lack of vitamin D has multiple adverse health consequences. It is linked not just to cancer, heart disease and diabetes, but also multiple sclerosis, rheumatoid arthritis, dementia, pre-eclampsia, and even infectious diseases such as influenza[50] It therefore comes as no surprise that taking vitamin D supplements is associated with a lower mortality rate[51].

Vitamin D is undoubtedly the 'in' supplement, but with so much of the evidence coming from observational and lab research, it remains a cliffhanger that leaves us dangling until the final chapter is written. We need properly conducted RCTs, and the conclusion to the vitamin D story looks likely to come from the VITAL study. This is a large RCT investigating the effects of vitamin D supplementation at 2,000IU per day in the prevention of cancer, heart disease and stroke in US adults over 50, as well as exploring whether there are any effects on the other health outcomes that we've discussed in this chapter. Unfortunately, with the trial just getting started, it will be at least five to six years before we start to get some real answers. In the meantime, we can only side with the inescapable conclusion that having a low vitamin D level won't do you or your health any favours.

With the stakes this high, in the next chapter we'll show you how to stay ahead of the curve when it comes to your health, with our guide to achieving optimal vitamin D levels.

SUMMARY AND RECOMMENDATIONS

- Low levels of vitamin D are widespread and likely to increase the risk of many chronic and life-threatening health problems.

- Evidence suggests that rates of cancer, heart disease, diabetes and autoimmune disease could be lowered significantly if we have adequate vitamin D levels.

- The good news is that the levels needed to realize this benefit are the same as for bone health, which is above a minimum of 20ng/ml, and nearer to 30ng/ml.

- We still need concrete evidence from well-conducted randomized controlled intervention trials.

- Until more results come to light, the weight of evidence to date supports the use of an appropriate regime to safely raise your vitamin D levels. This is laid out for you in the next chapter.

CHAPTER 7
'D'-LIVERED

OVERVIEW

- When it comes to vitamin D deficiency, we're faced with a big problem. But what's the answer?
- Why eating more vitamin D rich-foods simply won't suffice.
- The role of 'safe' sun exposure during the summer months to boost your vitamin D levels.
- How to avoid vitamin D 'starvation' in winter with an appropriately dosed vitamin D supplement.
- Finally, how much is enough, and can you have too much of a good thing?

We've seen that vitamin D is an indispensable nutrient for our health. Its benefits are not confined simply to our bones, but span many aspects of our health, bolstering our ability to stave off a number of chronic illnesses. Low levels of vitamin D are endemic and are among the most pressing public health issues of our times. To us, it's simply unacceptable to do nothing, so in this chapter we give you the solution and explain how to boost your vitamin D levels into the desirable range for optimal health.

Let the sun shine

By now you're probably eager to jump aboard the vitamin D wagon. But much of what we've mentioned so far is about levels of vitamin D in the blood, measured in seemingly abstract 'ng/ml' units rather than how much you actually need to take in order to reap the benefits. So we're going to make some no-nonsense recommendations to ensure you know exactly how to get the right amount of vitamin D.

It is important to note that our dietary intake of vitamin D is severely limited – even if you eat relatively good sources, such as oily fish, eggs, liver, meat and fortified foods, you're still going to fall way short. Diet typically provides less than 10% of our vitamin D requirements, with more than 90% coming from exposure to sunshine[1].

Throughout the whole of our evolution, right up to the present day, our primary source of vitamin D has been sunshine – not food. Just four minutes of summer sun exposure to one quarter of the body (arms and legs) in a young white person can produce 1,000IU of vitamin D[2]. In recent decades, the enthusiastic implementation of sun-awareness campaigns, vociferously encouraging us to reduce our sun exposure and to slap on the sunblock, has ensured the contribution made by the sun to our vitamin D status has diminished massively.

> **i** Even in countries with warm, sunny climates, such as Saudi Arabia, the United Arab Emirates, Australia and India, one third to one half of children and adults have vitamin D levels below 20ng/ml[3].

We're not saying that sun exposure is always beneficial. We now know that the effects of sun exposure are cumulative, leading to skin damage and ageing over time. Worse still, ultraviolet radiation, the very stuff that stimulates the skin to make vitamin D, has been classified as a class 1 carcinogen[4] and is linked to over 85% of malignant melanomas[5].

> **i** In 2007, 58,094 people were diagnosed with melanomas of the skin in the USA[6], so over-exposure to the sun is definitely not recommended.

> **i** A study in sun-drenched Australia found that more than 80% of 'sun-smart' dermatologists had low vitamin D levels. In fact, their average vitamin D level was lower than that of the elderly patients in a Melbourne Hospital[7]!

> **i** Go out in the sun and you risk skin cancer, stay out of the sun and you risk a plethora of other serious maladies, which leaves us with a massive catch-22.

But what if there was a way to reap the benefits, while avoiding the pitfalls? Could we strike a deal with the sun? After all, isn't this the way intended by nature? As set out in a unified view by the British Association of Dermatologists, Cancer Research UK, Diabetes UK, the Multiple Sclerosis Society, the National Heart Forum, the National Osteoporosis Society and the Primary Care Dermatology Society, total avoidance of the sun is not the aim. On the contrary, it's fine to go out in the sun in the middle of the day without sunscreen for a few minutes, as this is all the time you need to make appreciable amounts of vitamin D.

> **i** As a rule of thumb, you can only make vitamin D in the sunshine if your shadow is shorter than your height.

It's important to remember that the exact time we can spend out in the sun varies from person to person, and it's up to us to know our skin and to let common sense prevail. The key is not to get sunburnt –

that's NEVER a good thing. Taking a 'little-and-often' approach is the best policy.

Factors Affecting Vitamin D Synthesis

Skin exposure	Greater skin exposure equals greater area available for vitamin D synthesis
Age	Vitamin D synthesis ability decreases appreciably with increasing age
Skin colour	Melanin absorbs UVB, so the greater the skin pigmentation, the more time needed to make vitamin D
Distance from the equator	The higher the latitude, the less UVB exposure for production
Sunscreen	Using sunblock as low as SPF15 can reduce vitamin D production by 98%
Season	Limited synthesis in winter at higher latitudes
Body fat	Vitamin D is taken up by fat cells, leaving less in circulation
Glass	Allows sun exposure, but absorbs UVB, so vitamin D synthesis is not stimulated (i.e. when driving)

There is another major glitch when it comes to relying on the sun for vitamin D. In order for the skin to start making vitamin D, a UVB wavelength in the range of 290–320nm is required. This means that if you live in more northerly latitudes, you effectively experience a 'vitamin D winter', where even on sunny days during the winter months, it won't be the correct UVB wavelength to make vitamin D. This is found to be the case under clear conditions in places above 51 degrees latitude, such as London[8]. Indeed, there is no UV radiation of the appropriate wavelength for making vitamin D in the UK between the end of October and the end of March[9].

In areas of high ozone, the effect is evident from latitudes of 40–42 degrees and above[8], so we're talking about cities in the USA such as

Omaha, Boston, Chicago, New York, and even sun-rich countries such as Spain, France and Italy. If you live in Boston, you will be unable to make vitamin D from November through February[10]. At 70 degrees north (Northern Canada, Russia, Norway, Alaska), the vitamin D 'winter' period can last as long as seven months[8].

> **i** We strongly caution against using a sunbed, as any benefits are outweighed by the risks of melanoma. An International Agency for Research on Cancer report found that tanning beds increase the risk of skin cancer by 75% for those who use them before the age of 35[11].

So, despite 'safely' topping up vitamin D throughout the summer, it's highly unlikely that you'll be able to sustain your vitamin D at levels we would consider desirable (at least 20ng/ml, and ideally closer to 30ng/ml) throughout the winter. From summer to the end of winter, vitamin D levels will typically drop by 6–12ng/ml[12] – enough to catapult someone from a sufficient to a deficient state. Which leaves only one option. For most people, a vitamin D supplement is required to get them through the vitamin D winter 'famine'.

Supplementation: how much do I need?

When it comes to vitamin D levels, we recommend a range of 20–32ng/ml to be maintained all year round. The reason for the lower limit should be blatantly apparent by now; the reason for the upper limit will be explained a bit further on. With 'smart' sun exposure we can achieve this range in the summer, but for those of us who experience a 'vitamin D winter' the big question is, how much do we need to supplement?

In the UK, 47% of adults don't even reach levels of 16ng/ml in the winter/spring, and 87% fail to reach the upper desirable level of 32ng/ml (in Scotland it's 92%)[13]. Even in summer, when vitamin D levels peak, a whopping 61% of people still fail to reach that upper advantageous target of 32ng/ml[13].

We've already seen that we can't look to UK health authorities to lead the way. In their view, there's no need for a recommendation for 'healthy' adults, and only 400IU is required for vulnerable groups, which is tantamount to putting a sticking plaster on a broken leg. We prefer to let real science be our guide. A study from Ireland calculated that, in order to be confident that most adults (97.5%) maintain levels above 20ng/ml during winter, a dose of 1,120IU per day is needed[14]. The recommendation would be the same in the UK to achieve these levels. The study indicated that, with sufficient sun exposure during the summer, this recommended intake would keep many people near the upper end of the desirable range (20–32ng/ml) all year round. This gives us a recommendation of about 1,100–1,200IU, taken as a daily supplement from the end of October until the end of March. For ethnic minority groups, who have consistent low sun exposure/extensive skin covering with clothes, supplementation can be taken all year round.

> **i** You may not find vitamin D supplements sold in doses of 1,100–1,200IU, but a 1,000IU does the job perfectly. Just take one capsule per day, then on one day of each week take two capsules (eight per week in total) and you will be getting an average ideal daily dose of 1,140IU.

Americans tend to fare a bit better than the Brits – on average they hit the lower end of the desirable range of vitamin D levels, at around 20ng/ml. This is a consequence of a more proactive approach from the population. Some 30% of men and 40% of women in the USA already take vitamin D supplements, whereas the corresponding proportions in the UK are a mere 13% and 20% respectively[13]. To make matters worse, unlike in the USA and Canada, milk is not fortified with vitamin D in the UK. Only margarine is fortified, but with very small amounts. This paints a better picture, but vitamin D measurements for the population in the northern US states are made during the summertime[15]. By overlooking the effects of the 'vitamin D winter', surely this inflates the levels and gives a false impression? The fact remains that many Americans still don't supplement vitamin D, and milk, despite being fortified, won't fill the holes that the lack of sunshine creates. Furthermore, the amount of milk people are consuming has steadily declined in recent decades[16], meaning that winter supplementation is also required in the northern US states and Canada.

The Institute of Medicine (IOM) appears to be somewhat miserly in its recommendations, advocating supplementation of 600IU of vitamin D daily, but only for at-risk individuals, with a notable absence of advice to supplement in winter for those who live in the northern states. And is 600IU really enough? The IOM deems 20ng/ml as sufficient, though this really should be the very bottom of the desirable range (20–32ng/ml), with maximum benefits being seen closer to 30ng/ml. A good rule of thumb is that for every 100IU of vitamin D you consume, your vitamin D levels are raised by 0.4–0.8ng/ml[17]. These effects are more pronounced if your levels of vitamin D are already low, and less if they are already higher. We could therefore expect the IOM recommendation to increase vitamin D levels by about 4–5ng/ml.

> **i** Vitamin D is seized and locked down by fat cells, effectively taking it out of circulation. The fat holds on to it and doesn't let go, even when it's needed[18]. It's been found that, for every 10kg rise in body weight, an extra 17% vitamin D is needed[19]. With 68% of the US population classed as overweight or obese, this may have important implications[20].

In polar contrast we have the recommendations by Osteoporosis Canada for all adults under 50 to take daily supplements of 400–1,000IU (including during the summer), and for the over-50s to take 800–2,000IU daily. Their recommendations are, if anything, a bit over-zealous, and based on the belief that 30ng/ml is the minimum vitamin D level a population should be achieving, whereas we would suggest it should be the upper end of the range.

As the USA typically experiences greater summer sun exposure and a shorter vitamin D winter (being at a lower latitude), an intake of 800–1,000IU is all that's needed for those living in the states that experience a vitamin D winter (at 41 degrees latitude and above)[21]. This will ensure people are above the 20ng/ml minimum and put many at the upper end of the desirable range.

For Canada, being at higher latitudes, a recommendation of 1,100–1,200IU, as for the UK, is more suitable. Also, unless you are in a high-risk group with little sun exposure, just like the UK guidelines, supplementation is only needed for the winter and early spring months. As we're about to see, when it comes to vitamin D, it is all about striking the right balance – neither too little nor too much.

Guidelines for Vitamin D Supplementation in Adults

	Winter (October–March)	Summer (April–September)
UK	1,100–1,200IU daily	'Safe' sun exposure
USA – 41° latitude and above	800–1,000IU daily	'Safe' sun exposure
USA – below 41° latitude	'Safe' sun exposure	'Safe' sun exposure
Canada	1,100–1,200IU daily	'Safe' sun exposure

> **i** Supplementation of vitamin D is in the form of D3 (cholecalciferol) and obtained predominantly from sheep's wool and sometimes fish oil. Vegetarians or vegans sometimes prefer to take the D2 (ergocalciferol) form, synthesized from plants.

> **i** Vitamin D is fat soluble, and so the efficiency of vitamin D absorption is dependent on the fat content in the gut. Supplements are best taken with a meal containing fat[22, 23].

Proceed with caution

Just as it's important to ask how much is enough vitamin D, so too we should ask, how much is too much? There are many passionate vitamin D advocates out there who recommend that everyone should be taking mega doses, as high as 5,000IU daily. Even some analytical labs, which have to be scientifically meticulous in their operations, are sending back reports to medical practitioners with recommendations that their patients should be in the 40–80ng/ml range. It is claimed that this is all perfectly safe, as there is no data to show harmful effects at these high levels. The trouble is, they look at short-term studies to assess safety (and even a few years is short term when we're talking about a substance required throughout our entire lives), and define adverse effects as overt toxicity. In their eyes, when it comes to vitamin D, it's a case of the more the better.

Our take on this is a bit different. It's important to appreciate that the way vitamin D works in the body is subtler, and the consequences of excessive amounts could be more insidious in the long term than just looking for an obvious toxic effect in the short term.

One of the big mistakes that people make is to simply view vitamin D as a straightforward nutrient, when it should be regarded as a pro-hormone. Indeed, it's by hormonal actions that vitamin D can influence almost every tissue in the body, and that's why it's of such great importance to our health. But like all hormones, it's best to keep it within a healthy or optimal range. Having too little puts our health in jeopardy, but so does too much.

History tells us that when we discover the benefits of hormones we have a tendency to get a bit over enthusiastic. Just think about HRT (hormone replacement therapy). Initially it was believed that boosting hormone levels was the elixir of life, yet as the side effects emerged, HRT failed to live up to the hype. Sure, women need oestrogen to build up bone and reduce osteoporosis risk, reduce menopausal symptoms, improve mood, cognitive function, skin appearance and cholesterol levels. It took many decades, however, before we realized the darker side of promoting high levels, as they also increased the risk of endometrial and breast cancer, heart attack and stroke.

The same can be said for the male hormone testosterone. We need the right balance for a healthy cardiovascular system, healthy bones, mood, libido, strength, lean tissue gain, and many other reported benefits besides. But if levels are pushed over and above a 'healthy' range we find that, over time, it can stimulate unwanted prostate growth, worsen sleep apnoea, cause adverse changes to lipid profiles and increase blood pressure. Likewise, there are a large number of people with low thyroid hormone levels whose health and quality of life are transformed when they are given supplemental hormones. In the opposite camp are those who have levels that are too high, leaving them feeling equally poorly, and who need medication to reduce their levels.

'D' zone

Thinking that vitamin D would be any different makes no sense to us. It will be argued that vitamin D is 'natural', as it comes from the sun, and that high levels are what nature intended. That argument just doesn't hold up. First, we know that excess sun exposure massively increases skin cancer risk, so nature is actually forcing us to restrict our exposure. Second, even if we do have a habitually high sun exposure, it doesn't raise levels to the dizzy heights touted by many vitamin D enthusiasts. In a study of surfers in Honolulu, with heavy sun exposure of nearly 30 hours a week, the average serum vitamin D level was only 31.6ng/ml[24]. How can this be? It looks like Mother Nature was smart enough to build in a defence mechanism that prevents us from overdosing on vitamin D from sunshine, as any excess simply gets metabolized into non-active forms[25] (a defence mechanism not evolved for supplementation!). You can see that it's a pretty balanced system, designed to maintain a delicate equilibrium, which makes us fundamentally question the wisdom that 'more is better'.

As the research stacks up, some early warning signs of potential adverse effects from too much vitamin D are slowly emerging. Data from the third NHANES study in the USA suggested that those with vitamin D levels less than 20ng/ml had a 28% higher mortality rate than those with 30ng/ml or above. Although the correlations were only weak, every 4ng/ml rise in vitamin D levels was linked to a 7% reduction in mortality rate[26]. So, at first glance you'd be forgiven for thinking that 30ng/ml is the minimum you should target, and probably aim to go that bit higher. But if we look at the results in more detail, this is slightly deceptive. As vitamin D levels increased, mortality rates reduced until entering the 24–30ng/ml range and then started to creep back up. So those with levels above 30ng/ml had a 28% lower mortality rate than those with levels below 20ng/ml. However, those with levels of 24–30ng/ml had a 17% lower mortality rate than those with the levels above 30ng/ml. So it would appear that a mid-range level is optimal. Now, we need to point out that these were not very robust findings and on their own contribute only limited evidence, but they do proffer food for thought and contribute to the growing body of evidence that is emerging to caution us about getting over enthusiastic when it comes to supplementation.

Another study of women in the NHANES found that raising vitamin D levels to above 50ng/ml conferred no extra benefit, and there was a strong chance it increased overall mortality to as high, if not even higher, than those who were deficient[27]. Put simply, what this means is that both a deficiency and an excess of vitamin D are bad for us, so we should be aiming for the 'zone' in the middle, where we get all the benefits but none of the risks. This is exactly what was shown in a study looking at vitamin D and prostate cancer risk, which found that having both a low vitamin D status (<8ng/ml) and a high vitamin D status (>32ng/ml) was associated with higher prostate cancer risk[28]. A vitamin D level of 40ng/ml or above has also been linked with greater risk of pancreatic cancer[29]. And likewise, associations between higher vitamin D levels and oesophageal cancer have also been noted[30].

Undoubtedly, vitamin D is a complex nutrient which has the potential for both benefit and harm. However, this shouldn't distract us from the fact that vitamin D deficiency is endemic and that our levels are desperately in need of a boost. Rather, we must learn from the past and not be over-exuberant. As early as the 1930s lab research linked high oestrogen levels and HRT to cancer development, and the body of evidence started growing, but this was ignored and the reported benefits jubilantly embraced instead. It took nearly half a century before it was realized that the risks were serious. Learn from these mistakes, make note of the similar early warning signs coming through from research, and recognize that vitamin D needs to be treated with the same respect as all other hormones.

Just underway is the VITAL study, which is investigating the effects of 2,000IU supplementation of vitamin D in the US population (with the population allowed to consume up to another 800IU from other sources). We strongly suspect this will confirm that too much vitamin D may be as harmful as too little. Where this brings people into the optimal range, we predict this will deliver striking benefits, but in those individuals whose levels go too high, we suspect the results will not be so impressive. So, until the results are published, we advise that no one should consume such levels daily unless under the supervision of a clinician who is testing blood vitamin D levels. 'Balance is the key' and addressing the issue of vitamin D deficiency may well be one of the greatest steps we can take when it comes to improving the health of hundreds of millions of people worldwide.

THE PARTING SHOT

Whichever way you look at it, there's a widespread deficiency of vitamin D across the EU and in swathes of North America. The human and financial costs are vast. The benefits of achieving higher levels of vitamin D for bone health are now indisputable, and wider benefits for our health look increasingly likely. The great scandal is the fact that very little is being done about it. For sure, we need more rigorous clinical trials to confirm with certainty the observed health benefits of vitamin D. But, it's one thing to recommend restoring levels to a balanced range, and another to take a gung-ho approach to over-supplementing. The great thing is that the range proven to bolster bone health is exactly the same as is needed for the host of other associated benefits we've described. So, ironclad evidence or not, these are all bonus features of this essential hormone.

A case of our wellbeing crumbling as health authorities fiddle, it's up to you to take charge, and ensure you're in 'D' health zone.

SUMMARY AND RECOMMENDATIONS

- It's virtually impossible to obtain optimal intakes of vitamin D from foods sources alone – the sun has always been our primary source.
- Excessive sun exposure, however, and especially getting sunburnt, dramatically increases the risk of skin cancer and should always be avoided.
- Adequate vitamin D can be obtained in the summer months from 'safe' sun exposure – 'little and often' is best – combined with the use of supplements, especially in the winter months, to meet the body's vitamin D needs.

- The 'magic' level for vitamin D in the body is in the range of 20–32ng/ml. This is where the sum of the benefits has been observed to peak, and going above or below this level is associated with ill effects.

- A daily dose of 800–1,000IU in the USA, and 1,100–1,200IU in the UK and Northern Europe during the winter months is recommended for most people to maintain vitamin D levels in the desirable 20–32ng/ml range.

- You don't need to supplement in summer if you are getting regular 'safe' sun exposure, or in the winter if you live below 41 degrees latitude.

- Daily intakes should not exceed 1,200IU per day unless a clinician is monitoring your levels through blood testing.

PART III
DIET DISCREPANCIES

'In the middle ages, they had guillotines, stretch racks, whips and chains. Nowadays, we have a much more effective torture device called the bathroom scale.'

STEPHEN PHILLIPS, POET AND DRAMATIST **(1864–1915)**

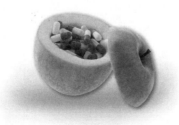

CHAPTER 8

FAD DIETS: A PACT WITH THE DEVIL?

OVERVIEW

- A burgeoning obesity epidemic means that 'dieting' has become part and parcel of many people's daily lives.
- How the mighty have fallen. We dissect the demise of the most popular diet of them all, Atkins.
- Popular diets have one thing in common – they're all fundamentally flawed.
- We uncover the true effects of dieting and why short-term success turns into long-term failure.
- Finally, we reveal the damaging legacy of dieting on metabolism, which scuppers future attempts at weight loss.

Recent decades have witnessed an unrelenting succession of high-profile fad diets. Each one bursts onto the scene with a flurry of publicity, and an obligatory celebrity endorsement, on its inexorable rise to the top of the bestseller book list. But look beyond the name, the celebrity icon, the pseudo-scientific claptrap, and you're left with pretty much the same thing – empty promises.

Debate continues to rage over which weight loss diet is best. The 'high protein, low carb' movement has been massive, inaugurated by Dr Robert Atkins with the mantle taken up by its less extreme successors, the Zone Diet and the South Beach Diet. Then there are others, fervently claiming the exact opposite to be true, such as the Ornish Diet, which trumpets a 'low-fat, high-carbohydrate' mantra. Of course, we have the enduring stalwarts too, such as the perennial Weight Watchers programme, a more middle-of-the-road affair focusing on calorie/point counting rather than specific macronutrient intakes. We could go on... and on... and on...

> **i** The diet industry's claim to fame is that we continue to get fatter. In the USA today, 68% of the population is overweight or obese.

A flawed concept

The truth is that it really doesn't matter much which dietary approach you choose. Despite new-fangled or pseudo-scientific jargon like the 'hormone zone' or 'ketosis', they're all designed to work in exactly the same way – you eating less. While they might promise that you can eat as much as you like, the simple truth is this: 'the laws of thermodynamics' aren't changing any time soon.

> **i** A calorie is a calorie and to lose weight you have to burn more energy than you take in, it's as simple as that!

As we're about to see, these diets are ultimately founded on a flawed principle. While they can proudly boast an initial weight-loss success, it is short lived. Not only are the effects transient, there's also a high price to pay. In the long run, there's a very high probability that the initial hard-earned weight loss will be regained, probably with added interest. And if that wasn't bad enough, there's a nasty sting in the tail because, as a result of dieting, you are now likely to gain weight faster and easier than ever before.

> **i** Obesity increases the risk of many health problems, such as the metabolic syndrome, type 2 diabetes, hypertension, coronary artery disease, stroke, cancer, reproductive dysfunction, osteoarthritis, and liver and gallbladder disease[1].

Low-carbohydrate diets

Without further ado, let's take this opportunity to drill down and have a look at the daddy of all weight-loss diets, Atkins.

Atkins is the archetypal high-protein, high-fat, low-carb plan. The diet entails eating unrestricted amounts of meat, cheese and eggs, but severely restricting carbs such as sugar, bread, pasta, and even fruit, vegetables and milk. The secret to success (apparently) involves 'switching our bodies from a carb-burning to a fat-burning machine'. This process is known as 'ketosis'.

And back in the diet's heyday, it looked as if Dr Atkins was on to a runaway winner, with astounding results being reported. Testimonials of people losing 6kg or more in a few short weeks were commonplace. Was this just hype? Well, even the scientific trials backed up the impressive anecdotes. In a study of 63 dieters, the Atkins diet was compared to the conventional low-calorie/low-fat/high-carbohydrate diet[2]. After six months the Atkins proponents were rubbing their hands with glee, it was a whitewash. The Atkins group had lost 7% of their body weight compared to a measly 3.2% in the standard diet group.

But here's the rub. After one year, the difference between the groups had narrowed dramatically (4.4% versus 2.5%). The initial advantage seen in the Atkins group ebbed away. The reason? The Atkins dieters regained nearly 3% of their body weight. The dramatic initial weight loss was simply a result of depletion of carbohydrate in the body.

Carbs are stored as glycogen in our muscles and liver, along with large amounts of water. Deprive the body of carbs and these stores become depleted. While this makes the numbers go down when you jump on the scales, don't kid yourself that this is fat loss. Thereafter, any subsequent weight loss is indeed real weight loss, caused by calorie restriction. Yet, despite the fact the Atkins group could eat high-protein or high-fat foods to their hearts' content, ultimately this still involved consuming less calories, and nothing more magical than that.

This was no one-off. In another study of 132 severely overweight individuals, a low-carb diet caused a far greater weight loss at six months compared with a low-fat diet (5.8kg versus 1.9kg)[3], however, at 12 months, these effects were diminished, resulting in little difference between the two diets (now 1.9kg difference)[4]. The popularity of the Atkins diet duly waned, as people realized its dramatic effects were short-lived, and that once the carbs were reintroduced the numbers on the scale started to move in the wrong direction again. Except for the most ardent dieters, it was simply too much effort for too little reward.

That's even before we add the potential side effects into the equation. The fact is we really don't fully understand the biochemical effects of such extreme changes to our diet. Despite gulping down all that saturated fat-laden meat and cheese, the Atkins Diet initially boasted improvements in traditional cardiovascular risk factors, such as cholesterol and triglyceride levels. Great PR for the diet, but surely this was too good to be true? It now appears that these initial conclusions could have been premature and naïve. In studies of mice, despite traditional risk factors not increasing, an Atkins-style diet caused levels of atherosclerosis twice that of a typical Western diet. This was due to dramatic increases in non-esterified fatty acids and decreases in endothelial progenitor cells, which are required to keep blood vessels damage free and healthy[5]. These are not measured in standard hospital cardiovascular testing, and so the initial clean bill of health for the Atkins dietary regime may be masking a ticking time bomb building up inside our blood vessels.

Other side effects of the diet included constipation, headache, halitosis, muscle cramps and rashes. These, on top of the cardiovascular worries, were enough to put the nail in the Atkins coffin. In 2005, the company filed for bankruptcy protection and, despite reinventing itself as a somewhat more carb-friendly and less-atherogenic version, it remains a shadow of its former self.

> **i** By 2004, such was the popularity of the Atkins Diet that it was estimated sales of the book had reached 45 million worldwide[4].

> **i** We can't blame the obesity epidemic on our genes. Obesity rates have trebled in a few short decades, which is far too quickly to be blamed on our genes. Obesity is driven mostly by our modern-day 'obesogenic' environments.

Short-term gains

Take a cursory look at the evidence on diets and you'll get the impression that they work pretty well. Let's take a RCT of 160 participants, evenly distributed to either Atkins (carb-restricted), Zone (high-protein, macronutrient balanced), Weight Watchers (calorie restriction) or Ornish (fat restriction) diets[6]. After one year, each diet had produced modest weight loss, with participants losing 3.9–6.6kg. (As an aside, we should mention the massive dropout rates – as high as 47% for the Atkins diet and 50% for the Ornish diet – which means if we factor in those participants who didn't finish the diet, the losses are more like 2–3kg.) Here's where it gets interesting. Maximum weight loss actually peaked at six months with a 5.2–6.7kg loss and by 12 months subjects had at best maintained, or worse, regained small amounts of weight in all groups. This was most notable in the Atkins group, which regained a whole 2kg (or roughly a third) of the weight loss seen at six months.

Let's look at a diet offering a so-called 'balanced solution', such as Weight Watchers. This programme is based on long-standing medical advice of restricting portion sizes and calorie intake, integrated with a group support system to improve compliance. In a well-conducted, multi-centred RCT of 423 overweight and obese individuals, the Weight Watcher programme resulted in a weight loss of 4.3kg after one year[7]. But again, here's the snag. At two years, this had reduced to a weight loss of 2.9kg. The participants had actually gained 1.4kg in weight during the second year of the diet.

These are not a few cherry-picked studies that we've selected to prove a point. It's easy to find short-term studies showing impressive weight loss, but all the long-term studies of dieting show the same thing: after six to 12 months the weight starts to go back on. As it happens, the Weight Watchers study was more successful than most, as the dieters did at least manage to lose a full 3kg in two years. But the sad reality is most long-term studies show that 80–90% of participants return to their starting weight[8]. All that hard graft and you're back to square one again.

> The annual turnover of the diet industry in the USA and Europe is in excess of a spectacular $150 billion[9]. It is ironic that the profits of the diet industry grow in parallel with rising levels of obesity. Clearly, the profits of this industry are not performance related!

Long-term costs

So, what's going on here? The proprietors of the diets would lay the blame firmly at your door. You are weak, you lack willpower and your initial good intentions and motivation, which brought about the early results, waned. They'll point to that rare success story of miracle weight loss (with obligatory 'before' and 'after' photos), as evidence of what proper commitment produces. Somewhere along the way you relapsed. Don't blame them, blame yourself.

We think it's high time that we placed the blame squarely on their shoulders, and to better understand why, let's take a look at one of the best-conducted RCTs of dieting that exists. A two-year study investigated various diets with different ratios of macronutrients in 811 individuals (80% of whom actually completed the study, which is impressively high for a diet trial)[10]. The macronutrients that were emphasized in each respective diet were protein, fat or carbohydrate, but it didn't make any noteworthy difference and similar weight loss was seen across all groups after two years, with participants losing about 4kg. What is important to note here, however, is that once again most of the weight loss was achieved after six months (on average 6.5kg) and after 12 months all groups started to regain weight. In fact, a mere 23% of participants, less than a quarter, managed to lose weight from month six to month 24.

Let's drill down to see what's going on here. At six months the groups were averaging a reduction of 400-plus calories from their starting point, with an intake in the region of 1,500–1,600kcals per day. This intake corresponded to a deficit of about 225kcals per day to lose 6.5kg after six months. At two years the participants were still averaging the 400-plus calorie drop from their starting point and, in fact, their calorie intake was slightly lower, in the region of 1,400–1,550kcals. Yet, surprisingly, this low-calorie intake was now causing participants to regain weight. For these participants, 1,400–1,550kcals now seemed to be a calorie surplus.

Bearing in mind that the recommended daily intake for adults is around 2,000–2,500kcals, the participants were not eating a particularly large amount. However, the damage caused by dieting meant that 1,400–1,550kcals had become their new daily 'set point' and if they were now to eat in excess of this pretty miniscule amount, they would gain weight. What was happening?

> **i** In 2002, a staggering 231 million Europeans attempted to diet. How many of those do you think were successful in achieving permanent weight loss? The unfortunate answer is less than 1%[11].

The body knows best

The truth is that the body isn't keen on us consuming low amounts of calories over prolonged periods of time. The human body is a primal machine that is highly adapted to getting us through times of food shortage and famine. Deprive the body of energy and it sends a clear message that food is in short supply. This sets in motion a signalling system to preserve our fat stores. It doesn't stop there either. The body won't get caught out so easily next time, so to 'future-proof' against any subsequent period of deprivation it creates more favourable conditions for energy (fat) storage. This mechanism has actually been known for more than 50 years and has been called the 'adiposity negative-feedback' model[12].

The body protects itself from food shortage in two ways. First, hormones are released, which act on the brain to increase appetite, thus making it harder to stick to a weight-loss diet. But most important is the second factor, which is called 'adaptive thermogenesis'. This is where the body dramatically reduces the amount of energy it expends in a 24-hour period. For example, let's say you lose 10% of your body weight by following a strict diet. This will reduce the amount of energy your body expends by 20–25%[8]. This reduction is far greater than would be expected simply from the decrease in metabolism from weight loss alone; its effect is over and above that. The upshot? A dieting individual will require around 300–400 fewer calories per day compared to an individual of the same body weight who has never lost weight. If that's not at least a bit shocking, check this out. These effects may not lessen over time. Dieting for even a few weeks appears to reduce energy expenditure persistently. In fact, these effects have been shown to last for years, with researchers concluding that they are very likely to last indefinitely[13].

THE PARTING SHOT

So that's it. Weight-loss diets might work initially, but for most of us, they will end up making us fatter in the long run. Worse still, any future attempts to lose weight will be harder and more gruelling than ever before. Far from being the antidote to the relentless progression of obesity, en masse dieting is priming us for it. Instead of helping the nation to beat the bulge, the diet industry is fanning the flames.

SUMMARY AND RECOMMENDATIONS

- See 'fad' diets for what they are – fads.
- Dieting gives good short-term results, but don't be fooled as the initial 'quick win' is usually short-lived.
- Diets start to backfire after six to 12 months and, despite dieting, the weight starts to creep back on.
- Depriving the body of energy for prolonged periods of time causes primitive mechanisms to kick-in to preserve body fat and 'protect' the body from further weight loss, thus making any future attempts at weight loss more difficult than ever before.
- Ultimately, fad diets of any kind aren't the solution to this oversized problem and in the next two chapters we'll reveal what does work.

CHAPTER 9
THE AGE OF THE SLOTH

OVERVIEW

- Is greed really to blame for the obesity epidemic?
- We shift our focus to the massive changes in our physical activity levels in recent decades and find them to be in terminal decline.
- Whereas dieting is doomed to failure, increasing our levels of physical activity is the key to slowing, and even reversing, the obesity time bomb.
- We look at how the effects of physical activity are not just limited to successful weight loss, but essential for promoting long-lasting health, too.

Now that we've exposed the fallacy of the fad diet, we want to deal with another canard. We hope you're sitting comfortably... deep breath, here goes...

The population is not meant to be cutting back on food because we don't have a problem with overeating. In fact, if anything, we are now eating less.

We know, we know. This is the 'fast-food nation', a population personified by gluttony, routine ingestion of a bonanza of calorie-laden drinks, fast food, sugary treats and supersized portions, all underpinned by an inability to know when we've had enough.

It's hard to argue with this. After all, the message to 'eat less' has been relentlessly drummed home. But the fact is, the science just doesn't back it up. A report from the UK Department for Environment, Food and Rural Affairs found that the 'average energy intake per person was at least 20% lower in 2005–2006 than in 1974'[1]. This is despite obesity rates more than trebling since the early 1970s. Figures for Canada from 1970 versus 1998 show a similar trend of increasing obesity paralleled by a notable overall decline in calorie intake[2].

A review of US national surveys found that the number of overweight people increased by 31% between 1976 and 1991, but calorie intakes were down 4% due to a rise in low-calorie food consumption[3]. Admittedly, this is at odds with the large NHANES study of the US population, which found that between 1971 and 2000, calories increased by 7% in men and 22% in women[4]. But the thing you need to know about these stats is that the jump in intake took place in the 1988–1994 survey period, when the survey was changed and questions added to get more complete answers, including – for the first time – calorie intake over the weekend. Considering that weekends are a common source of binge eating – on Saturdays we eat an average 12% more calories[5] – a reported increase is hardly surprising. Americans weren't eating more, the measurements were just getting better!

If we look at children and adolescents in the USA, there was no overall increase in calorie intake over the whole 30-year period[6]. Yet this is a population showing rapid rises in obesity, setting the stage for detrimental health impacts in adult life. China is also showing an alarming trajectory of weight gain. Once considered one of the world's leanest populations, it now contributes a fifth of the world's overweight and obese[7]. Yet surveys show that between 1989 and 2004 calorie intake has actually decreased consistently across cities, suburbs, towns and villages[8].

We admit that this might be hard to swallow, especially as it's been etched into our psyche that we're just a greedy and gluttonous bunch who have munched our way into this sorry predicament. Still, the data is hard to refute; as nations we're consuming the same or fewer calories than we were before rates of obesity soared. We should point out here that we're referring to the population as a whole, and clearly there are some individuals who are eating too much. But take a step back and look at the bigger picture. It tells us that the blame for the bulging belly of the majority can't be pinned on gluttony.

Lazy days

So, if calorie intake hasn't increased in recent decades, how has calorie expenditure fared? The fact is that we're much less active now than we were. Society has undergone remarkable changes and so has the way we go about our lives. The age of technology, for all the advances it has brought, has meant physical activity has been virtually factored out of our daily lives.

The things that have made the biggest dents in our energy expenditure include a decline in physical and manual work (now only 10% of men and 20% of women are in active occupations), and a greater reliance on motorized transport with corresponding reductions in walking and cycling (in 1952, the UK population cycled 23 billion km, compared to 4 billion km today)[9]. Add in common labour-saving devices, the use of lifts and escalators instead of stairs, and our choice of sedentary leisure activities (we now watch 26 hours of television a week compared to 13 hours in the 1960s), and we can see the 'age of the sloth' permeates every facet of our daily lives[9]. And while the individual changes appear trivial enough, add it all up and we get a shocking statistic: the difference between the activity levels of living 50 years ago and today is the equivalent of running a marathon a week[9]. And with that comes an incredible number of calories we are no longer burning.

Technology is great. We use it and we wouldn't want to be without it (and we're guessing you wouldn't either). But unless we actually want to, we really don't have to bother with the whole business of expending energy. We can roll out of bed, drive to work, take the elevator, sit at a desk all day, drive home, eat pre-prepared food, watch TV before rolling back into bed again, then do the same the next day, and the next.

The physical activity effect

It's not difficult to see that for all its good, technology comes at a price. By effectively factoring physical activity out of our day-to-day lives, it paves the way to obesity. There's a good deal of evidence that backs this up, too. A study of the EU member states found that active people were 50% less likely to be obese, and that obesity was strongly associated with a sedentary lifestyle and lack of physical activity, supporting the view that 'a reduction in energy expenditure during leisure time may be the main determinant of the current epidemic of obesity'[10]. Then we have the NHANES study (1971–1992), which examined factors influencing cardiovascular mortality in the US population. Its intriguing finding was that 'those who were obese and reported the least physical activity had the lowest caloric intake'[11]. This tells us that eating less doesn't guarantee you'll be slim, and eating more doesn't necessarily mean you'll be overweight. What does matter is the amount of physical activity you do.

A study published in the prestigious medical journal *The Lancet* found that changes in activity levels of US girls during adolescence had a significant effect on changes in their BMI and fat levels. But was it more important than what they ate? The authors concluded that, while activity levels played an important role in determining weight gain, energy intake did not exert the same effect[12]. It's yet more evidence that physical activity is the trump card. In fact, a dose response relationship exists between exercise and fat loss. When sedentary individuals begin a regular exercise programme, the more they exercise, the greater the amount of weight – and fat – they lose. Without any changes to diet, just one hour of moderate-intensity exercise, performed three days per week, could halt and even start to reverse the tide of obesity[13].

With this type of evidence, we don't think it's unreasonable to speculate that physical activity is protective against developing obesity, and that the dramatic declines in physical activity in recent decades go a long way to explaining the parallel rise in obesity.

Current rates of physical activity

Minimum recommendations state that we should be doing 30 minutes of moderate physical activity five times a week, or vigorous activity for 20 minutes, three times a week, or a combination of the two[14]. Such levels are associated with a multitude of health benefits, including reduced risks of cardiovascular disease, stroke, hypertension, type 2 diabetes, osteoporosis, obesity, colon cancer and breast cancer. Moderate-intensity exercise for more than three hours per week reduces the risk of mortality by an impressive 27%, while vigorous exercise of 20 minutes' duration three or more times per week reduces mortality risk by 32%[15]. Mortality rates are more than 50% lower in those who meet both recommendations[15]. A dose response effect is observable, and increasing your physical activity levels above the minimum recommendations will confer even greater benefits. It is recommended that, ideally, we should try to do up to one hour of physical activity per day for additional calorie burning and health benefits[16]. Don't think that the effects of exercise are limited to physical wellbeing, either. Studies show that regular exercise promotes better sleep, reduces depression, boosts self-confidence and increases our sense of wellbeing[17].

> **i** To obtain the health benefits of moderate physical activity, a minimum of ten minutes of continuous activity is required. In other words, you can't count the one- or two-minute walk to and from the car, even if you do it a few times a day.

> **i** The talk test is one of the best ways to measure intensity. If, during your activity, you can speak three or four words per breath, you are working at a moderate intensity. If you can only get one to three words per breath, you are most likely exercising at a vigorous intensity. If you can sing during your activity, it's not intense enough to realize health benefits.

Yet, despite all these highly desirable effects, surveys show that less than half of adults in the USA[18], and 39% of men and 29% of women aged 16 and over in the UK[19], say they meet the minimum recommendations for physical activity. And if these figures aren't bad enough, they actually paint a rose-tinted picture of the truth. When physical activity levels were objectively measured with an accelerometer, it was found that people were just kidding themselves. The figures shrunk to 5% or less who were actually reaching minimum recommendations for activity levels in both the USA[20] and the UK[19]. We've become so lazy that we're now living in complete denial. Yet somehow we're still intent on blaming food intake for our weight gain.

> **i** Is it better to train moderately for longer or harder for less time? It seems more vigorous activity has greater benefits for cardiovascular disease and mortality, independent of the contribution to energy expenditure.

> **i** 'High Intensity Interval Training' looks set to be the next big thing. This involves doing several short bursts of high-intensity exercise (e.g. sprints) separated by periods of lower-intensity exercise (e.g. slow or moderate pace). The advantage is that you get all the benefits of a workout, but in a much shorter time.

The following table lists different activities and their average calorie expenditure per 30 minutes.

Activity	Calories spent in 30 minutes
Sleeping	30
Sitting watching TV	37
Sexual Intercourse	100–200
Driving	60
Brisk walk (6.5kph/4mph)	185
Jogging (9.5kph/6mph)	375
Running (11kph/7mph)	430
Walking up and down the stairs in your home	210
Cleaning (washing windows, sweeping floors, mopping, vacuuming, etc.)	130
Mowing the lawn	205
Cycling to work	270–300
Basketball, soccer, tennis, swimming, volleyball, etc.	300–350
Elliptical Rider or Rowing Machine	425
Playing golf	1,000 (for 18 holes)

It is also recommended that aerobic activity be accompanied by muscle strength training exercises, such as resistance training and flexibility exercises, at least twice a week. This helps to build and conserve lean body mass, assists with enabling long-term participation in regular physical activity and promotes quality of life. Although this type of exercise is typically associated with the younger generation, it is especially important for older people to engage in it, too. The old adage 'use it or lose it' rings true, and strength training should be undertaken to prevent the seemingly inevitable loss of strength, energy and vigour with age. Performed regularly, this type of exercise builds muscles and bones, improves coordination and balance and prevents falls. In fact, it is one of the best 'anti-ageing' strategies of all.

i If you perform resistance training and are consistently able to complete more than 10–12 repetitions and/or you do not need to take a break (one to two minutes) in between sets, then your intensity is too low and the resistance (weight) needs to be increased.

i Wolff's law states that bones will adapt to the loads they are placed under. This is why weight-bearing exercise is particularly important for maintaining strong bones and warding off osteoporosis. Examples of weight-bearing exercises include brisk walking, running, aerobics, tennis and resistance training.

i Strength training, when performed correctly, is now recommended to improve chronic conditions such as arthritis, diabetes, osteoporosis, heart disease, obesity and back pain.

Dieting or physical activity?

We've set out our stall and said that we don't think dieting and excessive calorie restriction is the way to go. But where dieting falls down, physical activity steps up to the plate.

In the previous chapter, we discussed 'adaptive thermogenesis', and the idea that the body can dramatically reduce the amount of energy it expends when it loses weight by calorie deprivation (i.e. dieting). If you remember, we said that losing 10% of body weight can reduce the amount of energy the body uses by 20–25%. Well, it turns out that the vast majority of this decline, some 85–90%, is attributable to what's called 'non-resting energy expenditure', or in simple terms, the body's reduced ability to burn energy during physical activity[21]. This is because the efficiency of the skeletal muscles improves, reducing the amount of calories expended, especially during low-intensity activity. However, by using exercise as a means of weight loss, we target this very problem, increasing our non-resting energy expenditure and thereby avoiding the 'banana skin' of adaptive thermogenesis. And when it comes to resting energy expenditure, it appears that there is no compensatory decrease from exercise either, so it's a 'win–win'[22, 23].

Physical activity trumps calorie restriction in other ways too. Weight loss caused by restricting calories reduces the levels of our active thyroid hormone, which has the knock-on effect of decreasing our metabolism (the rate at which the body burns energy). However, when the same weight loss is brought about by physical activity, this reduction in thyroid hormone levels doesn't occur[24]. Whereas dieting puts the brakes on our metabolism, correctly performed physical activity can actually boost metabolism, with the effects lasting for hours after we stop exercising[25–27].

If all that wasn't impressive enough, the benefits of exercise even extend to the regulation of appetite. While dieting causes a backlash from the body, releasing appetite-inducing hormones to encourage weight regain as part of the 'adiposity negative feedback' system, no such effect is seen from exercise, and compensatory increases in hunger or food intake do not occur after exercise[28].

A RCT was performed in obese individuals to investigate the effects of a 700kcal deficit per day induced by either exercise (one hour of brisk walking and/or jogging) or calorie restriction[29]. At three months, both groups had lost 7.5kg (about 8% of body weight), though the exercise group lost more fat. And while we know the net result of dieting is gradual fat gain seen from six to 12 months onwards, with exercise we see long-term sustained weight loss[30]. It is thus unsurprising that members of the US National Weight Control Registry – individuals who have successfully achieved long-term, significant weight loss (averaging 32.3kg at the six-year mark) – are very active physically, with 70% exceeding minimum exercise recommendations. Nor is it surprising that those who were the most successful at weight loss were the most physically active[31, 32].

Many studies suggest that exercise alone produces only modest weight loss. This is simply because insufficient exercise levels are undertaken to create a big enough calorie deficit. Meeting minimum exercise recommendations burns about 1,000 calories a week. For significant and sustained weight loss, the equivalent of six to seven hours of brisk walking, or three hours jogging (2,000–2,500kcals) per week is required[33].

So there you have it: the ability to lose large amounts of weight to match any diet, but without the all-too-familiar and inevitable weight regain that undoes all your hard work. Instead, you just get the accompanying 'side effect' of dramatic improvements in your health.

> **i** A great way to stay motivated in your physical activity regime is to set yourself attainable and relevant short- and long-term goals, and to reward yourself when you achieve them. Your success is dependent on setting goals important to you, and your desire to achieve them.

> **i** With the increased strength and fitness capacity obtained from exercise, we can progressively build up the intensity/duration of our activity and circumvent any stagnation in fat losses that may occur.

THE PARTING SHOT

The weight-loss industry has commandeered the snake-oil market in recent decades. With billions upon billions being spent on weight-loss 'solutions', this is seriously big business. Let's face it, there's not a whole heap of money to be made from telling people to increase their activity levels. It's not a patch on the PR generated by the newest wonder diet endorsed by a Hollywood superstar (ironically, someone who looks great naturally, and probably hits the gym for hours each day anyway).

Who wants to sweat it out on the treadmill when you can just eat a particular diet – and be in 'a phase' or 'the zone' – shedding pounds while you lie on the couch watching the soaps? Unfortunately, as we now know, these diets don't work. It's time to accept that the emperor isn't wearing any clothes and these zealously endorsed diets wreak havoc on our long-term wellbeing.

Lest our message be misconstrued, we're not saying that you can eat what you like. After all, this whole book is about eating well. But don't confuse eating an optimally healthy diet with 'dieting', and remember that long-term success requires permanent changes in lifestyle and physical activity habits, on top of a healthy, balanced diet.

SUMMARY AND RECOMMENDATIONS

- Contrary to popular belief, on the whole we're not eating more than we were 30 years ago – a time before obesity rates were an issue.

- We may not be quite as greedy as we think, but we are more lazy – life in the modern world means physical activity levels have plummeted to an all-time low, paving the way to obesity.

- As well as stemming the tide of obesity, increasing our physical activity has an enormous range of other benefits for our physical and mental wellbeing.

- Aim to meet minimum recommendations of 30 minutes of moderate physical activity five times a week, accompanied by muscle strength training exercises at least twice a week.

- If you are already overweight or obese, you will need to go above these exercise recommendations to create a big enough calorie deficit for a significant weight-loss effect.

- While you should avoid 'dieting', you still need to combine increased physical activity with an optimally healthy diet to reap full weight- loss and health benefits.

- It goes without saying that you should seek professional advice before starting on any exercise regime, especially if you haven't exercised for a long time or have a medical condition.

CHAPTER 10
THE SKINNY ON FAT

OVERVIEW

- How useful are classifications such as 'overweight' and 'obese' for us as individuals when it comes to predicting disease risk?
- When it comes to determining whether we run the risk of obesity-related diseases, it's where fat is stored that really counts.
- We ask some big questions – is thin best, and is it possible to be 'fat and healthy'? – and get some surprising answers.

In the last two chapters, we dealt with the usual suspects of diet and physical activity, and hopefully set the record straight on some important issues. True to the spirit of keeping the best till last, there's another dimension to this debate that we've kept securely tucked up our sleeves until now.

Here's the thing. We've got so wrapped up with aspiring to the 'ideal' body weight, that we've missed a trick. We've got hooked into thinking that it's all about the numbers on the scales. If the numbers are good, we're happy. And if they're not, it spoils our whole day. The big snag with this sort of thinking is that we've got the 'ideal body weight' confused with the 'ideal body'. When it comes to our weight, it's really not all about the numbers on the scales. In fact, let's question the unquestionable, and challenge the very idea that thinness necessarily goes hand-in-hand with health and beauty.

What does it mean to be fat?

Back in 1970, Scott and Law attempted to define the morbidly obese:

> When an obese individual attains the gargantuan level of the fat man or fat woman in the circus, and maintains this degree of massive obesity for many years, we believe the adjective morbid should be added to emphasize the serious health implications and severe, life-shortening hazards of such grotesque accumulations of fat.

Forty years on, while the language we use to define excess weight has (thankfully!) progressed, we still find ourselves questioning how relevant these definitions are.

The most common measure used to define people as either underweight, a healthy weight, overweight or obese is Body Mass Index, or BMI. It's a simple calculation worked out on the basis of your height and weight (you can calculate it by dividing your weight in kilos by your height in metres squared). A BMI of 18.5–25 is the standard 'healthy' weight range, whereas 25–30 is 'overweight' and above 30 is classified as 'obese'. So, to show you how it works, a 60kg woman with a height of 1.65m, has a BMI of 22 $[60 \div (1.65)^2]$, which is classed as ideal.

For working out averages in a population, BMI is a very helpful device because it's quick, inexpensive and gives a general calculation. But when it comes to individual measurements, BMI lacks sensitivity and is a bit vague. To illustrate our point, you may have the same BMI as someone else, but you may also have twice the amount of body fat. Or, you may be a muscular rugby or gridiron player, but according to your BMI, you are classified as 'obese'. You can see that when it comes to individuals, looking at a simple weight to height ratio can be pretty misleading.

> **i** Wladimar Klitschko, a world heavyweight boxing champion, is 1.98m tall and weighs in at 110kg when competing. His body mass is 28, which classes him as overweight! Indeed, over half the England rugby team would be classed as obese, based on their BMI. We don't want to be the ones to tell them that they need to lose weight!

Not all fat is equal

There's also another glitch. We know that having increased body fat is associated with a significantly increased risk of many diseases. But there's an intriguing anomaly, as we will soon see. Numerous studies have found that this is not always the case. How could they go against the grain of one of the most established health principles of our times? Well, the thing is, it's not the amount of fat per se, but the distribution of fat that confers risk of disease. It's *where* we store fat that really counts, which explains why traditional measures, such as body weight and BMI, can be grossly misleading.

In 1947, Jean Vague coined the terms 'android' and 'gynoid' to define the two commonly observed body shape types – the 'apple' and 'pear' shapes respectively – suggesting that these different shapes conferred different health risks. Since then, it has become well established that it is abdominal obesity (android) that is associated with increased risk of cardiovascular disease, diabetes and cancer. For example, data from the large-scale EPIC study showed that abdominal fat was significantly associated with mortality risk, independent of BMI[1].

So, along came a new measure for being not just overweight, but also at risk of disease – a straightforward measurement of waist circumference. Based on that, it's now recommended that women and men keep their waist circumference below 80cm (32in) and 94cm (37in) respectively. The trouble is, it turns out that this is still a bit too simplistic and can be misleading. Not all fat is equal, and fat stored around the middle consists of two types of fat. There is the superficial and deep subcutaneous fat tissue (in effect, the 'surface' fat), and then we have the visceral fat tissue, the stuff that gets packed around our organs and spells trouble.

Here's where things get interesting. We tend to think that fat, or adipose, tissue is just a place where we store excess energy – a bit like a big storage depot. It just sits there, inert and benign, not doing much at all thank you very much. We couldn't be more wrong! Fat tissue is metabolically active. It manufactures and releases a host of hormones and pro-inflammatory chemicals that have been coined 'adipokines'[2]. And it's these chemical 'nasties' that are believed to confer the detrimental effects on our health of being overweight. Where do most of these adipokines come from? Visceral fat. This explains why it's visceral fat that is linked to the greatest risk of breast cancer, hypertension, raised cholesterol, diabetes and inflammation[3–5].

> **i** The Guinness World Record for the largest waist belongs to Walter Hudson of New York. In 1987, he measured in at 302cm (120in) – 30cm (12in) more than the record for the world's tallest man. He died just four years later, aged 46.

> **i** The corset was a popular fashion choice in the nineteenth century, giving the appearance of a slim waist. Wearers often suffered shortness of breath, movement restriction, weakness, digestive problems, fractured ribs, uterine prolapse and displacement of the liver. Still, this didn't deter them from their ideals of looking good no matter what, and many women wore a corset even during pregnancy.

The skinny fat

We all know one. And most of us are probably guilty of feeling more than just a twinge of jealousy towards them. It's that person. You know, the one who can eat whatever they want, never exercise, yet never put on a single pound... ever. We want what they have, but what is it? Good genes? A fast metabolism? A gift from God? Whatever it is, we want it.

But what if we told you that person might not be so lucky after all? What if their indomitable body could be a ticking time bomb, with no warning until it's too late? While it may not show on the outside, it's possible that their organs may be engulfed in visceral fat, which is sending out a deluge of noxious chemicals. Welcome to the phenomenon of the skinny fat.

Professor Jimmy Bell specializes in molecular imaging at Imperial College London. Using MRI technology he performs 3D internal scans of the body, which show how body fat is distributed. He found that 14% of men and 12% of women who are of 'healthy' weight according to their BMI, have significant excesses of visceral fat[6], putting them unwittingly at risk of all the obesity-related diseases. And who might we find among the ranks of the 'skinny fat'? Professional models, no less[7]. And one of the greatest risks for having a high visceral fat level, regardless of BMI, was brought about by following fad diets to lose weight.

If you've got the cash, there is another way to the so-called 'perfect body', and that's surgical removal of fat stores. The American Society of Plastic Surgeons reports that in 2010, 203,000 liposuction procedures were carried out, making it the fourth most popular cosmetic surgery in the USA. Liposuction, however, only removes fat from the subcutaneous layers. The dangerous visceral fat, with all the risks it entails, remains untouched. Undergo this procedure believing it's the cure for obesity and its related health risks, and you're in for a shock. In fact, it has even been suggested that in those with high visceral fat, it's possible that subcutaneous fat may actually offer some protection[8].

> **i** Fat distribution may have more than just physical effects. In an observational study of 16,325 females, those with the hourglass shape tested smarter and had smarter children. The authors suggest that such body fat redistribution contributes essential fats to neuro-development[9].

Fat and fit?

The effects of exercise on reducing our visceral fat stores and improving our health are truly dramatic. In the last chapter, we described the health benefits of being active. And we know now that physical activity ameliorates the health hazards associated with obesity, regardless of a person's overall weight or BMI[10]. In 2008, the results of an examination of 5,440 US adults were published[11]. They measured a range of risk factors for disease, including metabolic parameters such as blood pressure, triglycerides, glucose levels, inflammation levels and cholesterol profile, and uncovered some surprising results.

The prevailing assumption that being overweight or obese is automatically associated with bad health just didn't ring true. Half of overweight people (BMI 25–30) and one third of obese people (BMI >30) had healthy metabolic profiles, with blood results that didn't show them to be at increased risk of disease. And here's the twist. For nearly one quarter of the 'healthy weight' individuals, their results showed metabolic abnormalities that suggested increased disease risk.

What on earth was going on? What factors could begin to explain this disparity? We're sure you've guessed already: one of them was physical activity levels.

Let's look at it another way, by checking out a study that examined individuals who had similar BMIs and waist circumferences[12]. To the naked eye, the slim would undoubtedly look similar, trim and healthy, and the overweight, all fat and unhealthy. Where they did differ though was in their levels of physical activity. All the overweight individuals had similar amounts of fat and the same waist size, regardless of whether they were fit or not. But here's the important bit. After an MRI scan it was found that the overweight and unfit had nearly twice as much dangerous visceral fat as the overweight and fit. A similar trend was also found in the fit versus unfit slim individuals.

Fitness is the key

Fitness is a massive predictor of mortality. In a study of 21,925 men over eight years, those who were lean and unfit had twice the mortality rate of those who were lean and fit[13]. A 12-year study of adults aged over 60 suggested that the death rate of the unfit was more than three times that of those who were fit[14]. Fitness was measured by a treadmill endurance test, and all it took was to increase the time by about five minutes to cut mortality risk in half.

Considering the well-known health benefits of exercise, should we really be surprised that individuals who are fit are healthier than their unfit counterparts of the same weight? Perhaps more shocking is the repeated finding that individuals who are fit and overweight have lower rates of diseases and mortality than unfit 'healthy weight' individuals[13-16]. These results are especially apparent in the mild to moderately overweight category, where it appears perfectly possible that you can be 'fat' and healthy. So you see it all comes down to your visceral fat levels, which ultimately determine your true risk of chronic disease.

Let's take the most extreme example: the Sumo wrestler. A typical Sumo wrestler would have little problem in meeting the criteria for 'morbidly obese'. While we may think that their extraordinary bulk is incompatible with health, it appears that they are in fact metabolically healthy. Their physical activity levels mean that, despite their excessive calorie intake (a staggering 6,000–7,000kcals per day), their visceral fat levels remain normal. The problems arise when they retire and the ensuing lack of physical activity means bad health rapidly encroaches upon them.

> **i** A study of 5,000 UK women, average age 29, commissioned by *New Woman* magazine illustrated the extent to which image disfiguration has become engrained in 'normal' society, as 97% of respondents deemed that a UK size 12 (US 10) was 'fat', and 60% expressed desire for a UK size 2–4 (US 0) figure. One third had tried to maintain an extreme 500kcals per day diet in an effort to reduce their dress size.

> **i** Some people are just 'naturally' fit, but this doesn't get you off the hook. You may perform well in a fitness test, but irrespective of this, your lack of physical activity means you still run all the risks of ill health[12].

Back to exercise

We hope it is now clear that it's not just about what the scales say, or where you are on a BMI chart, your waist measurement, or even how you look. It's all a bit more complicated than that. But the good news is that the solution is a simple one. We need to get out and exercise. Being active will burn those visceral fat stores. Ignore that at your peril. Being inactive for just a few months dramatically increases visceral fat stores, and with that comes sizable increases in metabolic disease risk, such as deterioration of cholesterol profile and impaired insulin sensitivity[17]. The flipside is that engaging in just moderate exercise – 30 minutes or more, five times per week – prevents this accumulation.

Don't be fooled into thinking that you have to pound the treadmill for hours on end, or perform the physical feats of an Olympiad to get these benefits. Regular, run-of-the-mill, moderate activity will do just fine. Any sport or physical activity you enjoy (enjoyment and exercise don't have to be mutually exclusive!) is suitable. It's about day-to-day things too, like taking the bike instead of the car. Or getting off the bus a stop earlier, or simply parking further away to increase the distance you have to walk. Take the stairs instead of the elevator. Go outside and do some gardening. Play with your kids in the park, or get out more with the dog. Performed regularly, and at a moderate intensity, anything that has you up and moving will start to burn the calories and reduce those visceral fat stores.

Above all, don't fall into the trap of judging the success of physical activity purely in terms of numbers on the scales. It can be pretty de-motivating if you're putting in the effort but not seeing the end result. Even in the absence of weight loss, there'll be improvements on the inside that you can't easily observe on the outside, notably the all-important reduction in visceral fat.

While short-term dieting studies also show reductions in visceral fat, we now know the pitfalls that lurk there. Besides, in complete contrast to exercise, dieting will also reduce muscle tissue. When the weight goes back on, it gets stored preferentially as fat first, ultimately conspiring to make our visceral stores bigger than ever.

THE PARTING SHOT

It's not our intention to give a carte blanche to obesity, or to suggest that people can eat as much or as badly as they like, as long as they exercise later. That would be pretty foolish and it's not what we're saying. It remains an inescapable fact of life that there are far more overweight people who are unhealthy, than slim people who are unhealthy, and the heavier a person becomes, the more apparent the health risks. The bottom line is that being overweight and being inactive are both bad for your health. Either way, the solution is the same. Increasing levels of physical activity will bring about improvements in both.

For exactly the same reason, we need to challenge the belief that 'thin is best'. Looks can be deceiving, and when it comes to these issues, society seems to be moving backward. Some people in positions of influence may treat it with contempt, but the hourglass shape of subcutaneous body fat distribution is quintessential of the healthy female form, and surely superior to our aspirations for the contemporary skinny look, indifferent to how it is achieved. So bogged down have we become in ill-conceived perceptions that we've missed the forest for the trees.

Society needs to change, and the responsibility for that rests firmly on the shoulders of health authorities, health professionals, the media, the weight loss and fashion industries, and our culture itself. We doubt that will be happening anytime soon, so our message is a simple one: get active or pay the price.

SUMMARY AND RECOMMENDATIONS

- While both have their purpose, don't be fooled into thinking that your body weight or your BMI tells you everything.
- Not all fat is equal – it's the distribution of fat that dictates your risk of disease, notably the amount of 'hidden' visceral fat.
- Visceral fat is bad news because it releases a host of noxious inflammatory chemicals, which increase susceptibility to chronic diseases such as heart disease and cancer.
- Looks can be deceiving and it's perfectly possible to be thin on the outside but fat on the inside.
- Based on the same principle, the opposite is true – if you're fit, it's possible to be fat and metabolically healthy.
- It all boils down to getting more physically active – do that and you'll melt away that visceral fat and reap the health benefits.

PART IV
ANIMAL ATTACKS

'What I dream of is an art of balance…'

HENRI MATISSE, ARTIST AND LEADER OF THE FAUVIST MOVEMENT
(1869–1954)

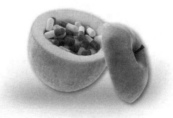

CHAPTER 11

WHAT'S THE MATTER WITH MILK?

OVERVIEW

- What's happened to the reputation of milk, the staple drink of our childhood?

- Why do so many people shy away from dairy products, believing them to be the cause of two of our most common cancers, prostate and breast? We uncover the evidence, which paints a rather different picture of milk.

- Rather than cancer causer, could milk be a cancer protector?

'Milk has gotta... lotta bottle, milk has gotta... lotta bottle, milk has gotta... lotta bottle, nice cold, ice cold milk!' went the slogan of the UK Milk Marketing Board's 1980s TV commercial, which put milk back on the map. Promoted as a health food, milk was suddenly cool to drink. 'It's got minerals and vitamins, to keep a body fit' we were told, and if the ads were to be believed, it was the favourite drink of sky divers, astronauts, racing drivers, and, for reasons unknown to us, women who enjoyed writhing around in shiny catsuits. But it seems the tide has turned in recent years, with our penchant for milk and dairy products undermined by the popular 'health' press. The anti-milk brigade tell us that milk is the cause of a whole host of diseases, with breast cancer and prostate cancer topping the list.

We weren't so sure it all stacked up, so we went on a mission to take a closer look.

'The China Study'

Let's kick off with a classic example, *The China Study*. This highly influential and bestselling book indicts animal-based foods as being the root cause of our so-called Western diseases. Its message is clear: avoid all animal-based products or face the consequences. The most persuasive (or should that be terrifying?) argument for avoiding animal-based foods is their purported effect of increasing the risk of developing cancer. To cut a long story short: if cancer were a fire, animal products would be the matches, the kindle and the fuel.

Well, that got our ears pricked up and we imagine yours too. There are no prizes for knowing that our modern-day diets lack plant foods: fruit, vegetables, wholegrains, legumes, nuts, and so on. Nor for thinking that if we dropped some of the meat products we consume with such gusto in favour of more plant foods, we would reap the benefits from ingesting more beneficial phytochemicals. We've no bones to pick with any of that.

But this wasn't the message being promoted. It was that animal products themselves, especially dairy products, were in the dock and charged with causing cancer. Yet, since 2004, when *The China Study* was published, there's been a raft of scientific research on this subject. So we took it upon ourselves to examine the three main cancers discussed in *The China Study* – prostate, breast and colorectal – to see if the evidence really stacked up. Next time we opened the fridge and laid eyes on the milk, cheese and yoghurt, would we recoil from it in the knowledge that we were staring at the source of our demise?

ℹ The dairy industry is massive in the USA, and valued in excess of a colossal $35 billion for the dairy farmers. In California, one fifth of the entire state's gross income is from milk production. The top dairy processors (Dean Foods, Kraft Foods, Land O'Lakes, Schreiber Foods, The Kroger Co. and Dairy Farmers of America) alone boasted sales of $26.5 billion in 2005.

You do the maths

Dairy products have been singled out as a primary culprit in the inexorable rise of prostate and breast cancer in the modern world, and it seems as if pretty much every 'alternative' health practitioner has got it in for the white stuff. This is fuelled by the massive variation seen in the rates of these diseases across different countries. For prostate cancer, the incidence is about 80 times greater in the USA than in China[1]. It's not quite as extreme for breast cancer, but still somewhere in the region of four times higher in the USA compared with Asian countries[2]. The anti-dairy contingent put these differences down to the fact that dairy products are consumed in large amounts in the West, but are practically non-existent in traditional Asian diets. To put it bluntly, we may as well be ingesting poison.

If you take a look at some of the science, it's not all that difficult to find studies to back up the anti-dairy soothsayers. Let's take prostate cancer, which shows the most extreme variation between West and East. In a study of 42 countries, milk consumption was closely correlated to prostate cancer occurrence[3]. That basically means the countries that guzzle the most milk get the highest rates of prostate cancer. Likewise, when we look at evidence from a number of case control studies, the risk of prostate cancer was cited to be 70% higher in those who consume milk[4].

So, if you just looked at these associations and nothing else, you'd be right to suspect dairy as the most heinous of foods. And you'd have little trouble constructing an almost identical argument when it comes to breast cancer, too. The stats look even more incriminatory when you look at what happens when people migrate from an area of low risk to an area of high risk (say, moving from Asia to the USA). The risk shoots up and within just one or two generations, Asians adopt the high risk of their host country. This tells us that it's the environment, not genetics, that's driving the stats up.

However, it's simply bad science to compare and contrast countries in this way. Do we actually think that we can take two totally different cultures and pin the differences in disease onto one single isolated dietary factor? Sure, it does have some intuitive appeal. China's dairy consumption is more than seven times less than that of the USA[5]. And even these low intakes for China still represent almost a doubling of dairy consumption in the last decade, with the greatest increases seen in the rapidly expanding urban population (urban intakes are five times that of rural intakes)[5]. And the idea is bolstered when we see that at the same time as this increased dairy intake, there was a 20–30% increase in reported rates of breast and prostate cancer[6]. But does it really all add up?

The thing is, we're talking about very different ways of life here, and far more differs than just dairy intake (better screening programmes, earlier detection, starting menstruation at a younger age, delaying having children, obesity rates and use of hormonal medications are just some of the things that might differ in the USA compared with China). But, while it seems ridiculous to blame the whole disparity on dairy products, it is still very possible that they have some role to play. So let's shed some real light on this and see what the studies have to say.

> **i** Dairy consumption started about 7,500 years ago in Central Europe and, as a result, Europeans have evolved to maintain the lactase enzyme, which digests milk sugar, throughout life. In contrast, many 'nouveau' dairy cultures, such as Asians and Africans, haven't made this adaptation and are generally lactose intolerant in adulthood.

> **i** Genetic factors may account for up to 10% of breast cancer cases in the developed world – a figurer far too low to explain the large variation in risk seen across different countries[1].

Prostate cancer

It's time to broaden our net and see what else is out there. In 2007, a major review of the evidence on diet and cancer was reported by the World Cancer Research Fund[7]. Comprehensive in scope, this would proffer some seriously authoritative facts and figures when it came to assessing the risk of dairy products in relation to prostate cancer. The report found an average increased risk of 6% per serving of dairy products (a serving being about 250ml milk) per day, so while apparently modest, the finding was surely enough to strike concern into the hearts of the dairy-gorgers.

The reason for this, it was suggested, is the high calcium content of milk. In support of this, a meta-analysis found that the highest calcium consumers had a 39% increased risk of prostate cancer compared with the lowest calcium consumers[8]. Results of the EPIC study published in 2008 proffered further support for this finding. While it found that just yoghurt intake, not milk or cheese, was associated with prostate cancer, when you added up all the calcium derived from dairy foods, those with the highest intakes had an increased risk of prostate cancer of 18% compared with those who had the lowest intakes[9].

So, it seems it's not milk per se that increases the risk of prostate cancer, but the fact that it's laden with large amounts of calcium. The evidence appears to point to a threshold for calcium intake. Hit about 1,500mg or more per day and the risk of prostate cancer starts to really take off[7, 10].

And is that really so surprising? Time and time again, the nutritional literature shows us that an over-reliance on very large amounts of a single nutrient can end up being harmful. As for calcium, there's never any need to ingest 1.5g or more a day, regardless of the source. Indeed, the increased risk isn't likely to be caused by high amounts of calcium itself, but the imbalance these mega amounts create within the body. What we need to do is keep our calcium intake in balance with our vitamin D levels, and taking masses of calcium can start to unravel that delicate equilibrium. Considering we are already a vitamin D-deficient population, the high calcium intake simply puts the balance further out of whack, which is not good news when it comes to prostate cancer risk.

> **i** It's estimated that 43% of the US population (and a majority aged over 70) takes a supplement containing calcium[11].

> **i** While a typical adult male in the USA consumes about 1,250mg of calcium a day[11], in China the estimated intake is a meagre 388mg and dairy contributes only 4.3% to the average daily calcium intake[5]. In China, the primary sources of calcium are vegetables, beans and bean products, wheat and rice[5].

> **i** Men concerned about prostate cancer should avoid consuming more than 1.5g calcium per day. That amount of calcium would be found in just over 1 litre of milk (or equivalent servings of other dairy foods). But remember that calcium is also found in other foods, and in some supplements, too.

THE SCIENCE BLAST:
CALCIUM, VITAMIN D AND PROSTATE CANCER

There's an interesting subplot to all of this. Those consuming the greatest amount of dairy products, associated with an increased risk of prostate cancer, tend to live at higher latitudes. With less sunshine, that also means they are a population with the lowest vitamin D levels. This lack of vitamin D results in reduced formation of the active form of the vitamin (known as $1,25(OH)_2D$) by the kidneys. In this situation, ingesting large amounts of calcium sets off a signalling system that reduces the active $1,25(OH)_2D$ even further, reducing the body's defences against cancer and increasing cell proliferation in the prostate. This was borne out in a study that observed that calcium, which reduced active vitamin D formation, increased prostate cancer occurrence, whereas fructose, which increases active vitamin D formation, reduced prostate cancer risk[13].

Intriguingly, a US study published in 2005 found an association with increased prostate cancer risk only with low-fat milk consumption and not full-fat milk[14]. We should also point out that milk in the USA is often fortified with vitamin D, which is fat-soluble. That means the low-fat version will have more calcium, but less vitamin D availability; more evidence for the importance of vitamin D in this whole debate.

So, it looks like it could be the low vitamin D levels, rather than the milk or calcium, that are the real problem. If you're already deficient in vitamin D (which, as we know, is all-too common) a high intake of calcium will just exacerbate the problem. It all boils down to getting enough vitamin D.

To illustrate the point, we'll look at a study that gave a pretty high dose of calcium supplements (1,200mg per day) to men already consuming 900mg calcium a day from the diet[15]. Based on what we know so far, we might expect this to increase prostate cancer risk. But it didn't. What you need to know about the subjects in this study is that they already had ideal vitamin D levels (at 30ng/ml). Vitamin D was in plentiful supply, which negated any harmful effects of a high calcium intake. So while the researchers found that the subjects given the calcium supplements had lower levels of the active form of vitamin D, made by the kidneys, the prostate would still have been able to make its own active vitamin D because the body stores were ample. If they'd started off with much lower vitamin D stores, it would probably have been a different story altogether.

> **i** Nutrients work together. Taking calcium as an isolated supplement is linked with around a 30% increase in heart attacks[12].

Hidden hormones

Time and time again, we hear that milk is bad for us because of the hormones it contains. Specifically, it is insulin-like growth factor (or IGF-1 for short) that's taken the rap for increasing cancer risk. IGF-1 causes cancer cells to grow, and raised levels are associated with a 47% increase in prostate cancer in men[16] and a 233% increase in breast cancer in premenopausal women[17]. With milk raising IGF-1 levels by about 10%[18], it's no wonder that dairy products are eyed with such suspicion by some.

But the evidence just doesn't stack up. Studies support the idea that soy can help reduce the risk of prostate cancer[19], and evidence suggests that consumption of soy throughout life may offer some protection against breast cancer[20]. Indeed, it is invariably the anti-dairy contingent who vociferously urge that we dump the dairy in favour of soy-based products. Yet ironically, soy protein actually increases IGF-1 levels significantly more than dairy does, with the magnitude of difference more than twofold[21].

In reality, IGF-1, made in the body from Growth Hormone, is essential for health and is dubbed an anti-ageing hormone. The problem is that IGF-1 doesn't discern between healthy cells and cancer cells, so if cancer is present it will promote its development. Once again, this underlines why prevention is better than cure. The job of preventing cancer formation in the first place is down to factors such as eating an optimal diet, getting enough phytonutrients, selenium and vitamin D, staying physically fit and maintaining a healthy weight.

Breast cancer

Of all the popularized diets for combating breast cancer, going dairy-free is easily the most widely propagated. As is the case with prostate cancer, the soothsayers cast dairy products as some sort of demonic perpetrator in causing breast cancer. If you want to stay free of breast cancer, you're told to ditch the witch.

Again, we turn to results from the EPIC study to shed some much-needed light on this. Studying the dietary habits of well over a quarter of a million women, the results found no consistent link between dairy products and breast cancer risk[22]. Then we have some fascinating results from a meta-analysis of 18 prospective cohort studies published in 2011, which found that overall, dairy products reduced breast cancer risk by 15% in those consuming the highest amounts, compared to those consuming the lowest[23]. This effect appeared stronger for low-fat rather than high-fat dairy products.

What's pretty clear is that dairy products, especially the low-fat varieties, have unnecessarily been given a bad rap. We simply don't think the science justifies it. It gets even more intriguing when we look specifically at calcium, which is found abundantly in dairy products. Lab studies have shown that calcium has anti-proliferative and pro-differentiation effects on mammary cells (so basically, anti-cancer effects), and in rats it inhibited the development of breast tumours[24].

Obviously we need data from human studies too, and when 15 studies on calcium intake and breast cancer were pooled together, there was a 19% decrease in breast cancer occurrence in those with the highest levels of calcium intake compared to those with the lowest[25]. There we have it. One of the key nutrients found in dairy products actually seems to protect against breast cancer.

> **i** When we also consider the strong association of vitamin D with breast cancer, it reinforces the importance of ensuring that calcium intakes are balanced with sufficient vitamin D levels[25].

Milk – an anti-cancer food?

Which brings us nicely to our final point. Why is it we only ever hear about the bad stuff? You could be forgiven for envisaging dairy as a digestive death sentence, so vociferously is it denounced. The dairy-bashing crusade is unrelenting, and its disciples are unwilling to give dairy any kudos. Well, for once, we're going to give you the positive spin. When it comes to breast cancer, instead of causing harm, we've seen that low-fat dairy, if anything, appears to exert a beneficial effect. The case for colorectal cancer is stronger still, with little doubt that it does a power of good. Studies consistently show evidence of protection from dairy intake. A meta-analysis of 19 cohort trials, published in 2012, found a 17% reduction in colorectal cancer from a 400g per day intake of dairy products[26]. The association was strongest for milk, with a 200g serving per day reducing the risk by 9%.

When we add in evidence from RCTs, the case gets even stronger. These show that the calcium in low-fat dairy reduces colon cancer risk by decreasing epithelial cell proliferation and improving cellular differentiation[27, 28]. Calcium can also bind fats and bile, preventing their irritating actions on gut cells.

THE PARTING SHOT

When it comes to cancer, it's pretty apparent that dairy has earned an undeservedly negative reputation. It seems that mother knew best when she said, 'milk does a body good'. So, next time the fear-mongers inform you that you're downing gasoline for the cancer fire, just turn and give them that white-moustached smile. Not only does the evidence fail to stand up, but dairy products, especially the low-fat variety, can actually reduce our cancer risk. As with everything, there is no need for extremes. If intakes are balanced, we can only conclude that dairy should reclaim its place as part of a healthy diet.

Got milk? Yes, please...

SUMMARY AND RECOMMENDATIONS

- There shouldn't be a blanket ban on dairy products for fear of increasing cancer risk.

- For men concerned about prostate cancer, it would be wise not to exceed 1,500mg of calcium per day (remembering that calcium is found in a diverse range of foods, not just dairy products).

- Maintaining an optimal level of vitamin D (20–32ng/ml), as described in Chapter 7, will further reduce any adverse consequences of dairy products on prostate cancer risk.

- There is no evidence that dairy products have an adverse effect on breast cancer risk; if anything, low-fat dairy products look likely to be protective.

- The most promising finding is that dairy products, especially milk, protect against colon cancer.

CHAPTER 12

WHAT'S THE BEEF WITH MEAT?

OVERVIEW

- A high intake of plant foods is a healthy way to go, but is eating meat actually bad for us?

- Get the lowdown on recently published evidence that helps us better understand the link between meat eating and cancer risk.

- Understand how the type of meat you eat, and how you cook it, are decisive factors in determining just how good or bad meat is for your health.

- Dispense with the urban myths and understand how to reap the nourishment meat offers, while slashing its health risks.

'If animals were not meant to be eaten, they would not be made out of meat'. So goes an antediluvian adage for those with little tolerance for the vegetarian way of life. But vegetarian diets are now an increasingly popular choice. Obviously there are well-principled moral and ethical motivations for eating plants over animals, and we have total respect for that. One thing's for sure: we're not here to preach on moral issues – you can make up your own mind whether eating meat is right or wrong. We won't be going there. We'll be sticking to what we know, and getting to the bottom of whether eating meat is bad for us, and, if so, whether we should all be joining the ranks of the vegetarians for the sake of our health.

As early as 500 years ago, the Italian physician Gabriele Falloppio cited beef and salty and bitter foods as the cause of cancer. Fast-forward five centuries, and the debate rages on. Remember the prolific-selling *The China Study* in the last chapter, and its assertion that dairy products were fanning the flames of chronic diseases such as cancer? Well, meat doesn't fare any better. Which leads us to ask the simple question: is this beef with meat justified?

Meat and bowel cancer

There's a classic urban myth that's been knocking around for years that says something along the lines of 'We can't digest meat properly, so it just sits and rots in our guts'. Nice. In fact, the story gets more and more exaggerated and the last we heard was that red meat sits in the intestines for at least seven years! Now that's a lot of meat. It was after the death of John Wayne that the rumour mill really shot into overdrive. Supposedly, during his autopsy, two kilos, then later 9kg, 18kg and up to 36kg, of red meat faecal matter was found impacted in his colon. How about that for an image to put you off your steak dinner?

Do we even need to say it's a load of crazy nonsense? Can you possibly envisage that just one steak a week would mean that you have 350 steaks sitting in your intestines? Or that you can have kilos of red meat building up inside you and never notice it? It's blatantly ridiculous. Of course we can digest meat; after all, we've had enough practice over countless millennia. All this prattling absurdity detracts from the real issue, which is that, folklore aside, there is legitimate concern that meat consumption is linked with increased bowel cancer risk.

Red meat refers to beef, lamb, pork and goat. Processed meat refers to meat that has been preserved by smoking, curing, salting, or the addition of chemical preservatives, and includes ham, bacon, salami, sausages and hot dogs[1].

Let's take a novel approach, and see what the science has to say. A meta-analysis published in 2009 looked at the intake of animal fat in relation to bowel cancer[2]. It found no increased risk for each 10, 20, 30 and 40g increase in intake of animal fat. It also showed no increased risk for animal protein intake. If you take that at face value, you could happily conclude that meat is off the hook. But a closer look tells us that it's far from a done deal. As is so often the case with research into diet, the devil is in the detail, and in this case, it's red and processed meats that perform the role of the devil. The meta-analysis we've just mentioned didn't differentiate between different types of animal protein, rather it lumped them all together. On closer inspection of the broader evidence, we see a different story. Poultry has a neutral effect, while fish is seemingly protective. In stark contrast, red and processed meat consumption dramatically increases bowel cancer risk.

Bowel cancer is the third most common type of cancer in men and women, with around 390 new cases diagnosed each day in the USA alone[3]. If you want to tip the odds in your favour, it's time to wise up to the type of animal protein you eat. In short, you'd do well to watch your intake of red, and especially processed, meats.

In 2007, the World Cancer Research Fund, in collaboration with the American Institute for Cancer Research, determined that red meat is a 'convincing' cause of bowel cancer. After an exhaustive review of all the evidence available, they determined that eating 100g of red meat a day increases your risk by 29%[1]. That is the equivalent of eating just three 8oz steaks a week (or the equivalent in chops, roasts, burgers or mince). Put it like that and this sizeable increased risk starts to look a bit scary. For processed meat, it's a grimmer picture still. Eating just 50g per day increases your risk by 21%.

So what's the score? What is it about red meat that so clearly links it to the risk of bowel cancer? First, cooking meat at high temperatures leads to the formation of some noxious cancer-causing chemicals called hetrocyclic amines, aka HCAs. It's the browning and charring of meat that generates these nasties. The EPIC study found that the risk of colorectal adenomas was increased by 47% in those with the highest HCA intake compared to those with the lowest[4]. Adenomas are benign tumours that frequently become malignant. The authors of the study found that the high HCA intake corresponded to those whose cooking methods produced excessively browned meat (sorry BBQ enthusiasts, but you're the worst offenders).

> **i** Cooking meat at high temperatures by frying, grilling or barbecuing ramps up the formation of HCAs. Cooking at lower temperatures, such as stewing, boiling or poaching, minimizes the amount of HCAs formed[1].

> **i** As well as HCAs, there are also polycyclic aromatic hydrocarbons (or PAHs). These are also thought to be carcinogenic and are formed during grilling or barbecuing. They are created when fat drops onto a direct flame, which leads to PAHs sticking to the surface of the food[1].

Red meat contains a particularly potent form of iron called heme iron, which is also a contender for the increased bowel cancer risk seen in high red meat consumers[5]. This could also help to explain why an increase in bowel cancer occurrence is not observed in poultry eaters. Heme iron causes fat oxidation, which produces nasty peroxyl free radicals that can be toxic to our genetic material. The heme iron in red meat also induces production in the body of nitroso compounds, which are carcinogenic. It is the formation of harmful nitroso compounds from the nitrite preservatives in processed meats that explains the particularly marked association between intake of these products and increased risk of bowel cancer.

Meat and breast cancer

While our take on the whole red meat and bowel cancer issue is pretty clear, when it comes to breast cancer, the waters are distinctly muddy. In fact, the only conclusion we draw is that there is no conclusion. As soon as one study is published saying one thing, another is published saying the opposite. Put simply, we have no definite answers on this one.

Take 2009, which looked like it would be the year the puzzle finally got solved. This was when the results of some of the largest trials investigating meat and breast cancer were published. It started in May, when the *International Journal of Cancer* reported the results of the 'NIH-AARP Diet and Health Study' cohort of 120,755 postmenopausal women who were followed for eight years[6]. The findings were pretty clear: a high intake of meat, including red meat, was not associated with increased risk of breast cancer. They looked at cooking methods too, and cooking at high temperatures, which as we now know produces a large amount of HCAs. Again the results showed no association with cancer incidence.

Just one month later, the *British Journal of Cancer* reported the results of the 'Prostate, Lung, Colorectal and Ovarian Cancer Screening Trial', which looked at the diets of 52,158 people[7]. Red meat was found to be associated with a 23% increased risk of invasive breast cancer, which appeared to be linked to its iron and HCA content.

Fast-forward three months to the September issue of the *American Journal of Clinical Nutrition*, and results from the 'EPIC' study were reported[8]. After following 319,826 women for eight years, the researchers were 'unable to consistently identify intake of meat, eggs, or dairy products as significant risk factors for breast cancer'. But there was an interesting side story. While there was no overall association of red meat with breast cancer, there was a lot of variation between different countries. Further investigation found that those countries that predominantly used high-temperature cooking methods showed red meat consumption to be associated with a 16% increased risk of breast cancer for each 150g per day, but this link was not evident for low-temperature cooking.

Just as a link was beginning to emerge, the 'Swedish Mammography Cohort' results were published in November[9]. Here, following 36,664 women for 17 years, no association between red meat or processed meat intake and risk of breast cancer was found. Back to square one. At the end of 2009, we were left more confused than ever.

When it comes to red meat and breast cancer, on the whole the evidence doesn't stack up in any convincing way. There may be no smoke without fire, but in the courts of science, innocent until proven guilty stands and the jury needs to be 95% confident to find the defendant guilty. Especially when we consider that meat eaters are more likely to be overweight[10] and on hormonal contraceptives[11] – factors known to increase the risk of breast cancer anyway. It's all very ambiguous. For now, the onus rests with the scientific community to collect more evidence and see if a conviction is warranted.

Meat and prostate cancer

Despite what you might have heard, the evidence for a causative role for meat in prostate cancer has always been pretty thin on the ground, with evidence pointing to a possible role for processed meat alone. In the 2007 report on diet and cancer, the World Cancer Research Fund/ American Institute for Cancer Research concluded that there was 'limited evidence from sparse and inconsistent studies suggesting that processed meat is a cause of prostate cancer'.

Since then, more studies have been conducted. A 2010 meta-analysis of prospective studies found no association at all between red meat intake and prostate cancer[12]. While processed meat was associated with a 5% increase in risk, this was only a weak correlation and 'non-significant', which means it could easily have been down to chance and not a real effect.

Making meat safer

OK, so the prostate cancer link holds no water, the breast cancer association is distinctly murky, but the bowel (or colorectal) cancer link stands up and conveys worry. So how much meat is safe to eat, if any?

Well, those clever boffins at the World Cancer Research Fund put their heads together and came up with the recommendation that people who eat red meat should consume less than 500g per week (cooked weight) and consume very little, if any, processed meat. We should point out, however, that this is a bit of an arbitrary guideline, based on practicality more than science. It will only mitigate, not quench, the bowel cancer risk. It is one thing to advise against processed meat, a pretty noxious product made by human interference, but strike red meat off the menu altogether, and likely the only people who will listen are those who renounced the red stuff long ago. So a happy medium of 500g was chosen to limit damage, while still allowing you to consume your weekly 16oz tenderloin. Yet it has been calculated that once you go above 70g a week (a measly 2.5oz), you start elevating your bowel cancer risk[13].

> **i** When observing the guidelines it is worth noting that 500g of cooked red meat is roughly equivalent to 700–750g of raw meat[1].

We have to say, we're not too keen on this compromise. Don't get us wrong, we enjoy a good steak, but to pass off an arbitrary amount as a safe limit, with no further guidance, is quite lacking. For many, this may be incentive enough to reduce red meat intake, but we also know there are a lot of meat fiends out there who won't be stopping any time soon. So we're going to take up where the World Cancer Research Fund left off and describe some simple tips for how you can make that 500g limit a whole lot better for you.

Step one: reduce the amount of HCAs produced and you will reduce the cancer-causing potential of red meat. Marinating meat before cooking will dramatically reduce HCA formation, especially if the marinade is packed full of herbs and spices. Indeed, one study showed a whopping 88% reduction in HCA formation with a Caribbean-style marinade[14]. Then, how you cook it is key. Avoid cooking at high temperatures, which burn or excessively brown the meat (particularly barbecuing). It's better to cook meat at lower temperatures for longer – for example, a slow-cooked casserole would be spot on.

> **i** The simple trick of marinating will confer protection, but to really reduce those HCAs include some proven effective quenchers. Choose virgin olive oil instead of refined oils[15]. Add lemon juice, garlic, onions[16], and herbs and spices such as rosemary and turmeric[17, 18]. And when it comes to beer or wine, it's beer over wine every time[19].

> **i** Make your marinade from scratch. Researchers have noted that some commercial sauces (e.g. barbecue sauce) can increase HCA formation, possibly due to high fructose corn syrup or honey in the mixture[18].

Step two: stop iron activity. In the last chapter, we saw that just a 200g serving of milk per day is associated with a 9% reduction in bowel cancer, likely due to the beneficial effects of calcium on the cells in the gut. As well as this, calcium inhibits heme iron absorption[20], so by taking a dairy food such as a yoghurt or milk (preferably low-fat) with or after meals, or using a yoghurt-based marinade, you can help stop the deleterious effects of iron.

Step three: incorporate flavonoids into your dish of red meat. So get busy with all the trimmings. Go full on with the onions, big it up with a citrus-based marinade, have a nice cup of green tea, or indulge in some after-dinner dark chocolate – all foods that pack a flavonoid punch.

Flavonoids not only appear to prevent iron absorption[21], they also prevent activation of HCA compounds. In the EPIC study, where HCA and high red meat intake was associated with a 47% increased risk of adenoma development, this association was rescinded in those with a high dietary flavonol intake[4].

THE PARTING SHOT

A lot of folk are pretty quick to 'diss' red meat, and we have to admit that, of all the anti-animal-product fervour that exists, this is the one that actually stands up to scrutiny. But at the same time, let's not forget that red meat is actually a highly nourishing food. It chalks up points for its plentiful supply of protein, well-absorbed iron (notably important for young women, among whom iron-deficiency anaemia is rife), zinc and vitamin B12. Clearly we're not giving you carte blanche to scoff as much as you want. Red meat comes with its caveats, especially with regard to the risk of bowel cancer, but used wisely it can definitely form part of a balanced diet. Keep your intake moderate, follow the advice set out above, and there's no reason why you can't have your steak and eat it.

SUMMARY AND RECOMMENDATIONS

- Fish and poultry show no adverse effects on cancer risk and are nutritious inclusions in the diet, especially fish, which may even reduce your cancer risk.

- Red meat and particularly processed meat are more suspect, and have been strongly linked to elevated incidence of bowel cancer.

- For this reason, processed meats such as ham, bacon, salami, hot dogs and sausages should be kept to an absolute minimum.

- If you do eat red meat, keep your intake below 500g per week (cooked weight), following the advice of low-temperature cooking, marinating and incorporating dairy products to reduce HCAs and iron activity.

- Red meat is best consumed as part of a diet rich in plant foods, especially flavonoid-rich foods such as vegetables (especially onions), fruit (especially berries, apples and citrus fruits), green tea, red wine and dark chocolate, which further neutralize any harmful effects.

- Let's not forget that red meat is an excellent source of vitamins and minerals such as iron, zinc and vitamin B12, and can make a valuable contribution to your intake of these essential nutrients.

CHAPTER 13

CAN PLANT-BASED DIETS PROVIDE IT ALL?

OVERVIEW

- Touted as healthy, what's good about vegetarian-style diets?
- Although they are a whole lot better than bog-standard Western fare, diets that rely solely on plant-based foods can fall short of the mark.
- Understand the nutritional shortfalls commonly seen in people following plant-based diets that could undermine heart health, bone health, brain health, hormonal health and the immune system.
- Learn how to fill in the gaps in plant-based diets, and why carefully chosen animal-based foods can help give you the best of both worlds.

Compared to the average meat-chomping Westerner, vegetarians appear to be a pretty healthy bunch. The idea that vegetarians are all pale, anaemic and sickly is a load of bunkum, and a lot of the research conducted into the health of vegetarians indicates that they fare well. So that got us thinking: can we thrive on plant foods alone?

A glimpse at the evidence on the health of vegetarians certainly tells an impressive story. Overall, vegetarians have lower rates of heart disease, lower levels of 'bad' LDL cholesterol, less high blood pressure, less diabetes and less obesity[1]. If that isn't enough to get you excited about lentils, they seem to have lower rates of cancer too, and can even look forwards to greater life expectancy[1]. Authorities such as the prestigious American Dietetic Association are vociferous in their support of vegetarian diets, stating that they are 'healthful, nutritionally adequate, and may provide health benefits in the prevention and treatment of certain diseases'[2]. It seems that there are many virtues associated with the vegetarian life.

A 'SAD' diet

Are we really so surprised that vegetarians have such good health stats compared to those eating an average Western diet? Or should we rephrase that to those eating a rubbish diet? Indeed, the Standard American Diet, or SAD for short, leaves a lot to be desired (and we can easily include the UK here too). In a year, the average American reportedly wades through 13kg of French fries, 10kg of pizza, 10kg of ice cream, 240 litres of soda, and 10kg of artificial sweeteners[3]. In the year 2000, it was estimated that the average American consumed 32 teaspoons of added sugars per day[4].

This is in stark contrast to the foods that are more likely to crop up in the diet of health-conscious vegetarians, namely fruit and veggies, cereals, pulses and nuts. Our modern diet is woefully lacking the plethora of beneficial phytochemicals found in plant foods. If vegetarians are eating more of these foods, we should hardly be surprised to find they experience better health. We challenge you to read the next paragraph and argue against eating more veggie stuff.

You've heard it all before, so we won't go on about fruit and veg too much, but suffice to say, eating plenty of the stuff reduces the risk of heart disease, high blood pressure and stroke, lowers cancer risk and reduces diabetes, and just for good measure, helps to promote healthy bones [5, 6]. Next up, nuts. Full of 'good' unsaturated fats, antioxidants, fibre, vitamin and minerals, they are a recipe for a heart-friendly food if ever there was one. The risk of coronary heart disease is 37% lower in people consuming nuts more than four times per week compared to those eating them rarely or never[7]. Eating wholegrain cereals (such as wholegrain bread, rice and pasta, oats, and so on) appears to protect against heart disease, obesity, diabetes and cancer[8, 9]. As for legumes (beans, peas and lentils, etc.), their substantial soluble fibre content lowers LDL cholesterol and triglycerides, and in addition to their cardio-protective credentials, they may also protect against diabetes and obesity[10, 11].

Who would turn their nose up at such a who's who of health benefits? It doesn't really matter two hoots whether you eat meat or not; either way, you should be ditching the junk and including more of these foods. Enough said.

> **i** The Standard American Diet is typified by over-consumption of refined grains, sugars, trans-fats, fast foods, and high-energy-dense snacks. A truly 'SAD' way of eating that is fuelling the epidemic of chronic degenerative disease.

> **i** Vegetarians do not consume any meat, poultry, game, fish or shellfish, or by-products of slaughter, but can choose to eat dairy products and eggs. Vegans additionally avoid eating dairy products and eggs, and any other products derived from animals.

We would do well to bear one important fact in mind. Most of the studies into the health of vegetarians are epidemiological. Generally, that means taking a bunch of vegetarians and a bunch of non-vegetarians, and following their health over time to see what happens. Most of the time, the vegetarians come out on top, getting less disease. But these are only associations, they don't prove that it's the avoidance of meat that makes the difference. It's a pretty reasonable assumption that vegetarians might generally be a more health-conscious lot, with a range of healthy behaviours that make them different from their non-vegetarian counterparts. For example, vegetarians are likely to be slimmer, to smoke less, and to have a higher socio-economic status compared with the wider population[12, 13], and there could be any number of other subtle differences in behaviours and attitudes that aren't so easy to measure.

The point is: it would be a leap of faith to say with any certainty that the health benefits seen are down to not eating meat. There's a clever study, which recruited almost 11,000 British men and women, that illustrates this. The participants were either customers of health food shops, or people with an interest in health foods or vegetarianism. It's fair to say that they were all likely to be health-conscious individuals, but only 43% were vegetarians. The study found no significant differences in all-cause mortality, or mortality from heart disease or cancer, between the vegetarians and the non-vegetarians (in fact, the study actually found increased mortality from breast cancer among the vegetarians)[14].

Not so heart healthy?

So, what would happen if we switched to a diet that was made up of just plant foods? After all, the research tells us that these foods are the business when it comes to keeping us healthy, so why not just ditch the animal foods once and for all? Well, despite all their nutritional plus points, the bare fact is that plant foods struggle to provide some of the important nutrients that are simply much more readily available from animal sources.

With all that fibre, all those fruit, veggies and wholegrain cereals, and the lack of saturated fat, you'd think that a plant-based diet was the absolute daddy of all diets to prevent heart disease... well, not quite. Vegetarians, and especially vegans, can easily find themselves lacking vitamin B12[15, 16]. This might quickly undo the cardio-protective qualities of the veggie diet by raising levels of homocysteine, a toxic by-product in the bloodstream that is strongly implicated in heart disease, as well as a range of other diseases. Non-meat eaters have been shown to have higher homocysteine levels than meat eaters[16, 17], showing us that this is one area where plant-based diets fall down. We can only get vitamin B12 from animal foods (including dairy products and eggs), so eat nothing but plant foods and sooner or later you'll end up deficient. If you wish to eat a strictly plant-based diet, the only way around this particular conundrum is to regularly consume foods fortified with vitamin B12 (e.g. fortified soy or rice beverages, fortified breakfast cereals, fortified meat analogs, or B12 fortified nutritional yeast), or take it in the form of a supplement[18].

We're not quite done here yet. Plant-based diets are sorely lacking in another piece of the cardio-protective jigsaw – the long-chain omega-3 fats EPA and DHA. These are the types of omega-3 fats found almost exclusively in oily fish. They simply don't occur in plant foods, yet they're highly beneficial for cardiovascular health (not to mention brain health, and helping to control inflammation in the body). It is possible to get omega-3 from plant foods in the form of alpha-linolenic acid, found in foods like flaxseeds/flaxseed oil, walnuts/walnut oil and rapeseed (canola) oil. However, this is a poor man's version of omega-3 and lacks the clear health benefits associated with the more potent EPA and DHA. Now, in theory, the body can convert the plant form of omega-3, alpha-linolenic acid, into the more desirable EPA and DHA. The problem is that it's just not very efficient at it. The conversion of alpha-linolenic acid to EPA is about 8–20%, while to DHA is 0.5–9%[19]. The lowest conversion rates are seen in men, and women achieve the meagre but relatively higher end of the range. So, don't be conned by so-called nutritionists and supplement companies claiming that their plants and oils, such as flax, provide great sources of omega-3s.

The truth is that eating a purely plant-based diet leads to significantly lower levels of EPA and DHA. A study of British men found that, compared to meat eaters, EPA was 28% lower in vegetarians and 53% lower in vegans, whereas DHA was 31% lower in vegetarians and 59% lower in vegans[20]. Not only that, but the ratio of fats in typical plant-based diets tends to be heavily skewed towards omega-6, contributing to a decline in tissue levels of omega-3[21]. As you'll see in Chapter 16, an excess of omega-6 relative to omega-3 is not good news for our cardiovascular system, our brain, or for keeping inflammation in check.

> **i** It is now possible to buy supplements of DHA derived from algae. These are a suitable source of long-chain omega-3 fats for vegans and vegetarians.

A bone to pick

The two biggies when it comes to bone health are calcium and vitamin D. Vegetarians who consume milk and dairy products will do just fine when it comes to getting calcium. But the calcium intake from a purely plant-based diet, without any dairy products, can be pretty marginal[22]. When it comes to vitamin D, as you now know, deficiency is rife, but this is especially so if you shun animal-based foods. Admittedly, meaningful dietary sources of vitamin D are few and far between, but include oily fish, and, to a lesser extent, eggs and milk, so it's little surprise that plant-based diets fall well short of the mark[23, 24].

This should all be ringing a few alarm bells for bone health, and as might be expected, following an exclusively plant-based diet is associated with lower bone mineral density[24, 25]. In the Oxford cohort of the EPIC study, fracture risk was compared in 19,249 meat eaters, 4,901 fish eaters, 9,420 vegetarians and 1,126 vegans. While there was no difference among meat eaters, fish eaters and vegetarians, the vegans showed a 30% increased fracture occurrence, which appeared to be a consequence of their low intake of calcium[26]. While it is possible to get calcium from a plant-based diet, getting enough is hard work, and such studies underline the fact that plant-based diets struggle to make the grade when it comes to bone health.

> **i** Plant sources of calcium include low-oxalate green vegetables (e.g. kale, broccoli, Chinese cabbage, collards), calcium-fortified beverages (soya milk, rice milk, fruit juices), tofu set with calcium, sesame seeds and almonds.

Missing without a trace

Most dietary minerals are only needed in small, trace amounts, yet they have a big role to play in keeping us healthy. Some, such as copper and manganese, are abundantly available in a plant-based diet[27], whereas others can be in short supply. On one hand, minerals like iron and zinc are less 'bioavailable' from plant foods, which means the body just can't absorb and use them as efficiently. This causes concern that levels of these key minerals could be pretty marginal in a plant-based diet. On the other hand, plant-based diets can also lack other trace minerals, like selenium[28, 29], especially in a country like the UK, where the selenium status of the population is already low.

> **i** Vitamin C greatly assists with the absorption of iron from plant foods[30]. This can be achieved by consuming vitamin C-rich fruit/fruit juices and vegetables with meals.

> **i** Soaking and sprouting/germinating beans, grains and seeds can reduce the inhibitory effects of phytic acid, improving iron and zinc bioavailability[2].

Another good example is iodine. Very high rates of iodine deficiency (80% for vegans and 25% for vegetarians) have been found in people eating plant-based diets[31]. While universal salt iodization is an effective strategy for eradicating iodine deficiency[32], the UK is rock bottom of the international league table when it comes to availability of iodized salt[33]. Consequently, practically no one in the UK is using it, which means we're totally dependent on getting it from our diet. This comes from eating fish and seafood, and also milk. You can see where we're going with this – eat a diet of only plant foods without iodized salt, and you're likely to run into trouble. Why does all this matter? Iodine is vital for making thyroid hormones, which are absolutely critical in governing our metabolism. Failure to get enough iodine will compromise this, which as you'll see in Chapter 15, may have particularly severe repercussions in pregnancy.

> **i** Plant-based diets often include foods that contain substances known as goitrogens, such as soya, cruciferous vegetables, flaxseeds, millet and sweet potatoes. Goitrogens – which are inactivated by cooking – can interfere with thyroid function, especially when iodine intake is insufficient. So vegetarians are especially at risk, and getting enough iodine is crucial.

> **i** Seaweed is very rich in iodine; however, it can contain extremely high and potentially excessive levels[34]. Just as too little iodine is harmful to the thyroid gland, so is too much.

THE PARTING SHOT

If we put all the ethical and moral issues to one side and focus purely on the health aspects, we don't think there's a strong argument for eating a purely plant-based diet. The fact that a plant-based diet lacks so many really important nutrients suggests to us that it was never intended as the optimal diet for a human being. Sure, there are literally loads of benefits to be had from eating a diet rich in plant foods, especially given the funky array of phytochemicals they contain. Anyone eating the 'SAD' way would do well to urgently heed that message. But we reckon a plant-based diet gets even better if you supplement it with some carefully chosen animal-based foods. That's not to say that you can't achieve these benefits with a purely plant-based diet, but if that's your inclination, then you've got to give the whole thing a lot of thought and ensure that you attain all those missing bits by careful dietary choices and appropriate supplementation.

SUMMARY AND RECOMMENDATIONS

- Vegetarians generally experience good health, with less chronic disease and greater life expectancy. However, putting this down to the exclusion of meat is a premature conclusion.

- The benefits of a vegetarian diet have a lot to do with the consumption of a wide range of plant foods, which have well-documented health-promoting qualities and are sorely lacking from the standard Western diet.

- This means we should all be striving to eat a diet that contains plenty of plant-based foods, such as fruit and vegetables, wholegrain cereals, legumes and nuts.

- However, purely plant-based diets run a big risk of nutritional deficiencies, which could be counterproductive to the health of our hearts, brains, immune system, hormones and bones.

- Well-chosen animal-based foods, especially fish and low-fat dairy products, plug the gap perfectly.

- If you're committed to avoiding animal-derived foods, then having a carefully planned diet, plus appropriate use of nutritional supplements and fortified foods to provide vitamin B12, vitamin D, calcium, iron, zinc, iodine, selenium and omega-3 fats, will protect you against deficiency.

PART V
GENERATION GAINS

'Nobody can go back and start a new beginning, but anyone can start today and make a new ending.'

MARIA ROBINSON, CONTEMPORARY CHILD BEHAVIOUR AND DEVELOPMENT SPECIALIST AND AUTHOR

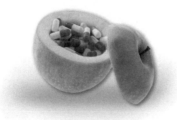

CHAPTER 14

YOU ARE WHAT YOUR MOTHER ATE

OVERVIEW

- Can the origins of disease be traced back to the womb?
- Did you know that your birth weight could be a powerful predictor of your future risk of numerous chronic diseases?
- We look at how rapid growth in the early years can predispose us to future illness.
- And we ask: could the first 1,000 days of life be the most important of all in determining our health and susceptibility to disease?

Medicine spends the vast majority of its time and effort treating serious illnesses that have typically been years, even decades, in the making. Whether it is type 2 diabetes driven by years of excess weight and sedentary living, the imperceptible loss of bone that culminates in an osteoporotic fracture, or the gradual silting up of our coronary arteries that finally results in a heart attack, this is where the mighty resources of medicine are deployed. As the growing burden of chronic disease threatens to overwhelm healthcare systems, we are rightly shifting our attention to prevention, for, as we all know, prevention is better than cure. We're implored to be more active, shed some kilos, eat our fill of fruit and vegetables, cut the salt and so on and so on.

But what if we've missed a trick here? What if the most critical time for preventing disease has long since passed? What if that was actually right back at our conception, and during the first 1,000 days of our life? What if our future health and susceptibility to disease was 'programmed' before we'd even taken our first breath?

A life mapped out?

A bit like outer space or the depths of the oceans, we are only just beginning to understand the 'environment' of the mother and how it affects the susceptibility to health and disease of the developing offspring. And just as we once thought the Earth was flat, so too have we had to have a serious rethink on this. As recently as the 1950s, it was commonly believed that the foetus was the perfect parasite. In similar style to the US Cold War stronghold built into Cheyenne Mountain, Colorado, it was believed to be impervious to outside stresses and attacks. There was just one way in: a tunnel with an impenetrable barrier that ensured what wasn't wanted stayed out. For the baby this tunnel is known as the placenta. Back then, we thought the placenta allowed the developing foetus to block all noxious substances, while preferentially taking up the nutrients it needed. The foetus looked after itself and all mum had to do was house it for 40 weeks. Just think, it was only a few short decades ago that it was commonplace for mums-to-be to regularly drink alcohol and smoke (in the 1950s about half of US mothers smoked during pregnancy[1]).

Of course, things are a bit different now. Hard lessons have taught us not to take such a lackadaisical approach to prenatal care. We're now fully aware that harmful substances, such as certain medications, recreational drugs, alcohol and cigarette smoke, can cross the placenta and wreak damage. Likewise, we recognize the need for good nutrition to ensure the birth of a healthy child (sufficient folic acid to prevent neural tube defects being a classic example). As long as our child is born healthy, and is seen to develop normally early on, the time in the womb was a success, right?

But what if we are still being too complacent about the potential of those formative months to mould and shape our health as adults? What if this period turned out to be the most critical time in our lives when it comes to disease prevention? What if our health throughout our entire life was predestined there, the blueprint of wellness (or lack of) laid down before we even took our very first breath? Perhaps that all sounds a bit far-fetched? But it's exactly what UK doctor David Barker of Southampton University has proposed. In 1986 he made the 'heretical' claim in a paper published in the prestigious *Lancet* journal that heart disease in adult life is 'related to nutrition during prenatal and early postnatal life[2]'.

The Foetal Origins Hypothesis

In the early 1900s the health of Britain was in a dire state. One in ten infants failed to see his or her first birthday, and those who did survive were often rife with maladies. In the national press of the time, it was claimed that up to two thirds of young men who volunteered to fight in the Boer War were rejected because of their unsatisfactory physique[3]. So worrying was this downturn in the nation's health that one medical officer described it as a sign of the 'doom of modern civilization as it did that of Rome and Greece[3]'. Then, something special happened, thanks to the dedicated work of a midwife, Ethel Margaret Burnside. Having persuaded the clerk to Hertfordshire county council to provide 60 spring balances, she set to work with her army of nurses, recording the weight of every baby in the county, both when they were born and again at one year of age[3]. This information was meticulously stored in ledgers and gave rise to the famous Hertfordshire Records. Decades later, it was here that the Barker/Foetal Origins Hypothesis was discovered.

With access to these records, Dr Barker was able to track down 15,000 men and women who were born between 1911 and 1930. He found that 3,000 had passed away, almost half from coronary heart disease or related disorders[3]. There was a striking finding. A disproportionately large number of these deaths had occurred among people who had been born underweight. Dr Barker's team found that those who had weighed 5lbs (2.25kg) or less at birth had twice as many fatal heart attacks as those who weighed more than 10lbs (4.5kg)[3]. It wasn't just about being born small, either. There was a change in risk right across the normal range of birth weights, meaning that as you move up through the birth weights, so heart disease risk in later life falls[4]. So if you were born 7lbs (3.2kg), you had less risk than if you were born 6lbs (2.7kg), and if you were born 8lbs (3.6kg) you had less risk than if you were born 7lbs (3.2kg). And it was with these eyebrow-raising findings that the Barker Hypothesis was born.

> **i** There's a limit to the benefits of a high birth weight. Mothers who are overweight and/or with diabetes going into pregnancy, or who develop gestational diabetes, are at risk of giving birth to high birth weight babies. As well as increased birth complications, these infants also have a greater predisposition to become overweight in later life[5, 6].

Later, a systematic review of 18 studies of 147,009 individuals examining birth weight and ischemic heart disease risk, found a consistent 10–20% reduction in risk for every kilogram increase in birth weight[7]. Similarly, researchers have calculated that a 100g increase in birth weight would reduce coronary heart disease deaths in later life by 2.5% in men and 1.9% in women[8].

What we're left with is a quite remarkable discovery. If you were small at birth you are biologically different and these differences stick with you for the rest of your life. Blood pressure is higher, levels of fats in the bloodstream differ, the artery walls are less elastic, the stress response is altered, as too are hormone levels, the risk of type 2 diabetes is amplified and ageing is accelerated[3]. In essence, the foetal origins hypothesis proposes that the effect of under-nutrition in early life alters the structure of the body and how it functions... permanently.

While we blame an unhealthy diet and lifestyle for many of our Western chronic diseases – such as heart disease, high blood pressure, diabetes and osteoporosis – could they actually be instigated during our time spent in the womb? Could it be that poor nutrition in pregnancy causes deleterious physiological changes that predispose us to these diseases in later life?

> **i** It's not just nutrition but other stresses that have a programming effect. When mothers smoke during pregnancy, birth weights are lower but infants are more likely to become overweight in childhood[1].

Programming

So what's going on here? How could something as apparently innocuous as birth weight exert such profound effects on the risk of disease decades later and with such unerring accuracy?

It looks likely that some adaptation occurs in the foetus during pregnancy in response to poor nutrition. From nine weeks post-conception onwards, the foetus starts to experience rapid growth. Different tissues grow at different times and these have been labelled 'critical periods'. Optimal growth and development of these tissues is dependent on an adequate supply of nutrients, and if this is not available, the growth rate slows down and the number of cells, and the structure of the organs, can be permanently altered.

> **i** The Barker Hypothesis is not about babies who are born
> prematurely – it is full-term babies born small because
> of restricted growth in the womb that are at risk.

But there's something else going on here too, something quite amazing. The low nutrient state of the mother acts as a signal to the developing child that the environment it will be born into is going to be a nutrient-impoverished one. The message is clear: you will be born into surroundings where food and nutrients will be scarce, so you'd better be prepared. As a consequence, what takes place is a 'programming' effect, thought to occur through hormone changes. The anabolic hormones IGF-1 and insulin are reduced and the catabolic hormone cortisol is increased. Cortisol is thought to be particularly significant here, exerting a growth-inhibiting effect on all tissues when the levels are raised in the developing foetus[9–11].

If you think about it, it's actually a very clever early warning system. The foetus is sensing its environment and based on this, is making predictions for the future – will it be born into a world of plenty, or will it be born into a harsh world of scarcity? Either way, it needs to be ready. If the latter is the case, this in-utero programming prepares the foetus for optimal survival advantage in an environment where nutrition is poor. In essence, a 'thrifty phenotype' is developed[12].

But what happens when this baby, primed for a nutrient-poor environment, is actually born into a world where food is plentiful – i.e. the affluent Western world? Suddenly, the programming is at odds with the environment. Alas, the 'window of opportunity' for 'programming' is now closed, and the 'lasting memories' have been created. With the baby's metabolism geared up to survive in nutrient shortage, the sudden exposure to plentiful nutrition means that nutrients are efficiently hoarded away as fat, serving as a store for any perceived future famines. Programmed at birth to conserve and store energy, yet bombarded with a lifetime of high-energy foods and a sedentary lifestyle, it becomes susceptible to the chronic diseases of our times – heart disease, obesity and diabetes.

Catch-up

If we're not careful, we can end up compounding this problem. If a child is born at a weight below the 'norm', our natural inclination is to increase its calories to encourage 'catch-up' growth. This has long been viewed as an essential feature of recovery from the possible ill-effects of restricted growth in early life. As we begin to better appreciate the 'thrifty phenotype', it looks increasingly likely that this is the very worst thing we could be doing. It might intuitively seem right to 'feed them up' if they are small, but by doing this, all we're actually doing is increasing their future risk of disease[13, 14].

So-called 'catch-up' growth in infants is consistently linked with increased fat mass, especially central fat, in childhood and adulthood[15, 16]. And with this comes the highest rates of blood pressure[17], heart disease[18] and, potentially, diabetes[19] in adult life. It seems we're not just talking about the first year or two either, but into early childhood. Infants who were born small and remained thin at two years of age, but thereafter put on weight rapidly, had insulin resistance and higher coronary events in adulthood[20]. What we're talking about here is not nutritionally depriving the infant – on the contrary, we need to be especially conscious of giving high-quality nutrition – but rather to avoid going overboard and giving excessive calories to try and rapidly promote growth back into the 'normal' range, as the infant is simply too susceptible to fat gain. As the infant grows into early childhood, this is a key time to really emphasize the promotion of a healthful diet and physical activity to negate any deleterious programming effects.

A 'natural' experiment

Despite the mounting number of supportive observational studies, and the convincing mechanistic and animal data, the problem is this may all just be circumstantial, and falls short of proving cause and effect. This was borne out by a meta-analysis of 110 studies investigating birth weight and later life blood pressure, which suggested there was too much random error and too many confounding effects to accurately illustrate the effect of the apparent association[21].

One of the big criticisms of this whole theory is that factors such as smoking or socio-economic class could act as major confounders, in which case the low birth weight is just a reflection of some other factor, and not a direct cause. So for example, if you are poor you are more likely to have a worse diet during pregnancy, leading to a lower birth weight. Of course, being in poverty doesn't stop just because you were born, it's likely to remain with you throughout all stages of your growth and development, and as we know, being less well off is generally associated with worse health outcomes overall. So maybe we're reading too much into the significance of a low birth weight when in fact it's just a reflection of levels of affluence.

If you could conduct any research you wanted to sort this out, then ideally you'd perform an intervention trial. You'd take a population of women trying to conceive, some rich and some poor, and divide them equally into two groups. You'd restrict the nutritional intake of just one of the groups during the pre- and early postnatal period, before returning them to their normal diets. Then you'd follow the newborns for life to see if those with the restricted nutrition ended up with more health problems like heart disease, obesity and diabetes. It would 'control' for socio-economic status and give you a pretty good idea of whether the whole foetal origins hypothesis holds true. The big problem with our study is probably obvious – it's completely unethical and would never be allowed!

But sometimes we're offered the next best thing – a 'natural' randomized intervention trial that is conducted courtesy of circumstances, as was presented by the Dutch Famine of 1944. During the winter of 1944–45 half of Holland was under Allied control while the other half was under German control. An embargo was placed on food transport into the west of Holland, and by the time it was lifted, frozen canals and other waterways ensured a state of famine with severely rationed food supply. Upon the German surrender in the spring of 1945, this state of starvation ended, and nutritional intake was once again unified across Holland. And by the fate of history, a 'natural' experiment was conducted. In a population of diverse socio-economic status, we had an experimental group (exposed to famine and thus a deprived nutritional status for a defined period of time) and a 'control' group (consuming their typical diets throughout). Which leads us nicely on to the big question: would the offspring of pregnant women from the famine group experience worse health than those in the well-fed population? Could exposure to low nutrition in the womb affect lifelong health?

The results were striking. Nutritional deprivation at any stage of pregnancy increased insulin resistance in the offspring[22]. When deprivation occurred early in pregnancy, greater heart disease, as well as an increased prevalence of obesity, was observed[22]. In the case of females, the risk of developing breast cancer in later life increased almost fivefold[22]. Interestingly, it was found that the programming of chronic disease that occurred wasn't always linked to a reduced birth weight.

This suggests that birth weight is just one obvious marker of under-nutrition, and that more subtle nutritional insults may occur which predestine future risk of chronic disease, remaining hidden until it presents in later life.

Indeed, the effects of under-nutrition encompass not just 'physical' disease, but mental health problems, too. A twofold increase in schizophrenia was reported in the follow-up of the offspring of the Dutch famine and also in a study of famine in China[23]. And perhaps that's only the tip of the iceberg. Low birth weight children demonstrate lower cognitive ability and attain fewer advanced educational qualifications[24, 25], as well as being less likely to be employed in later life[26]. Other studies have even shown that low birth weight individuals are less likely to get married[27].

What does it mean for us?

Of course, we don't really experience things like famine here in the developed world. But perhaps our problem is not a lack of food per se, but a lack of the correct foods. We have many women of child-bearing age who consume unbalanced junk-food diets high in sugar, salt and trans-fats, but deficient in key vitamins, minerals and essential fats. We may not be calorie deprived but many remain nutrient-deprived. It may be different from the chronic malnutrition we see all too frequently in the developing world, but it still results in poor nutrition for the foetus. A junk-food diet could be hard-wiring the next generation for disease.

The optimal development of the foetus is highly dependent on the delivery of appropriate levels of a spectrum of essential vitamins and minerals. A shortfall of these can impair tissue development and induce hormonal changes, and has been associated with a reduced birth weight[28, 29].

So, what does this contentious hypothesis mean for us? Do we sit back and just blame mum for our disease risk? While the arguments are compelling, we need to get it into perspective and remember that it is just one factor among many we experience throughout our lives that may increase or decrease our risk to disease. Not every 'programmed' baby goes on to develop disease. For most of us, it is better viewed as determining the degree of our susceptibility to the ill-effects of our environments, i.e. the poor diet and inactivity that defines our modern lives. By partaking in a lifestyle of proper nutrition and regular activity we can minimize the influence of this risk factor. For example, while the incidence of coronary heart disease was highest in women who were born underweight and went on to be overweight in adulthood[30], those who stayed lean into adulthood despite being born underweight had no observed increased risk. Your fate still remains in your hands, and whether you fulfil the plan imprinted on to you in early life is up to you.

> **i** If you were born full-term weighing less than 5lbs (2.25kg) – and possibly even 7lbs (3.2kg) or less – it becomes even more pertinent that you ensure you follow a healthy diet and lifestyle.

THE PARTING SHOT

The public health implications of this provocative hypothesis are potentially enormous. Rather than frantically firefighting the over-whelming burdens of obesity, heart disease and diabetes that we see all around us, should we be focusing our efforts on ensuring optimal nourishment during early life? Are we on the brink of a brave new world of medicine that prevents chronic disease before we've even taken our first breath?

Exciting as it sounds, it's all too easy to get carried with this. All we're doing here is bringing to light one more factor that may influence your health throughout your lifespan. It's the realization that any serious attempt at reducing the epidemic of chronic illness we face in the twenty-first century requires us to take a whole lifespan approach to health. Strategies for preventing chronic disease shouldn't start when we're in our 40s or 50s, but by our parents before conception, and then continued throughout all stages of life.

With that nailed, in the next chapter we'll move on to discussing exactly which key nutrients are needed, and at what levels, to ensure you give your child not only the best start in life, but also the gift of health that lasts long into adulthood.

SUMMARY AND RECOMMENDATIONS

- Chronic diseases such as heart disease and diabetes may not be all down to genetics and lifestyle – rather, our experiences in the womb, and during our first few years, could shape and mould them too.

- Poor nutrition in the womb can lead to restricted growth and permanent changes in the body that set the scene for chronic disease later in life.

- If we are serious about preventing disease, we need to ensure that future generations receive the best possible nutrition in-utero, and throughout early childhood.

- Optimal nutrition for women of childbearing age now, and especially during pregnancy, will help ensure that the next generation is a healthier one.

CHAPTER 15

NOURISHING THE NEXT GENERATION

Overview

- Getting the nutrition of the mother spot on during pregnancy presents a golden opportunity to shape the future health and wellbeing of the next generation.

- Understand how current dietary advice for pregnancy is mediocre, and missing some critical pieces of the nutritional 'jigsaw'.

- Many pregnant women are at high risk of missing out on key nutrients essential to the optimal development and health of their offspring.

- Failure to get these nutrients can increase pregnancy complications, impair growth and compromise mental development.

- With the right know-how, you can avoid these pitfalls by including the right foods and supplements in pregnancy to give your child the best start in life.

As we've seen from the Foetal Origins Hypothesis, our time in the womb can hardwire our future health. And if you just stop for a second and think about it, there's a big message for us here. What we have is a truly exciting opportunity to provide the next generation with the best possible start in life and to build a strong foundation for their health. Show us a parent on this planet who doesn't want that for their children.

Unfortunately, when it comes to dispensing this vitally important advice in pregnancy, it's a pretty pathetic effort. Sure, we get the usual sage advice to quit smoking, curb the booze, watch caffeine intake, eat a well-balanced diet (whatever that means for most people) and take a folic acid supplement – even though, as we'll see, for many pregnant mums, that particular piece of advice is given too late for maximum benefits anyway. This is all well and good, and we don't take issue with any of it. But all we're really doing is ticking a few boxes, and in the process missing out on a whole lot of other important ones that are also vital for the optimal development of your child during his or her time in the womb.

The nutritional supplement companies haven't missed this gap in the market, with their array of products 'tailored' for pregnancy. But in our opinion, these are often no more than a nutritional 'lucky bag' (many of the nutrients are unnecessary, and they even manage to miss out some of the important ones). Even the best of them, which do include the key nutrients that really do make a difference in pregnancy, are given in doses that lack scientific credibility.

Parents want to do the right thing by their children, so we'll take up the mantle and give you a rundown of the real nutritional needs for an optimal pregnancy.

Iodine

When it comes to nutritional messages for pregnancy, iodine is clearly the one that got away, receiving very little limelight in the UK and USA alike. That's all a bit worrying when we consider that iodine is absolutely vital for the developing foetus, as it has an indispensable role in thyroid function (it makes up 59–65% of the thyroid hormones in weight). Our thyroid hormones are essential for regulating our metabolism, and have a crucial role to play in the growth and development of organs, most importantly the brain. If you lack iodine, you run the risk of having low levels of thyroid hormones. And if that happens when you are pregnant, foetal development will be impaired.

So, it's the sort of nutrient that everyone needs in sufficient quantities. But you only need to look at the iodine levels of populations across the globe to see how deluded we are when it comes to our health. Over 2.2 billion people in the world are iodine deficient, making it the greatest single cause of preventable brain damage worldwide[1].

If you take a cursory look at women in the USA and UK, they seem to be doing okay with their iodine intake and are just about getting enough[2, 3]. But once pregnancy kicks in it's a whole different ball game. Requirements jump up to meet the additional need for sufficient thyroid hormones to satisfy mother and baby alike. While a normal adult needs 80mcg iodine per day for thyroid hormone synthesis, the greater metabolic demands of pregnancy increase this requirement to 120mcg per day[4]. And in pregnancy, the amount of iodine lost from the body via the kidneys actually increases by about 30–50%[4]. The upshot is that during pregnancy, the usual recommended intake of iodine of 150mcg per day is nowhere near enough – pregnant women need a hefty 250mcg per day[5]. The same amount is also needed throughout lactation, to ensure sufficient iodine is provided via the milk supply to the child.

When we apply these recommended levels for pregnancy to the US population, we see that a whopping 57% of pregnant women fall short of iodine[2]. The situation in the UK is similarly dire with about 50% of the pregnant population significantly iodine deficient[6]. Worryingly, a recent UK survey assessing iodine status in schoolgirls aged between 14 and 15 found iodine deficiency was present in over two-thirds of those sampled. In the not-too-distant future, it will be the children of these young women who will be most susceptible to the damaging effects of iodine deficiency, leading the authors to conclude that there was 'an urgent need for a comprehensive investigation of UK iodine status, and evidence-based recommendations on the need to implement a policy of iodine prophylaxis'[7].

> **i** The availability of iodized salt in the UK and Ireland is appallingly low – in fact, the UK and Ireland are firmly rooted at the bottom of the international league table when it comes to iodized salt availability[6].

Why does all this matter? The most damaging effect of iodine deficiency is seen in the first trimester of pregnancy, spelling big trouble for a baby's mental development. Iodine deficiency, or a lack of maternal thyroid hormones, is implicated in increased infant mortality, impaired growth, hearing defects, cretinism, impaired neurodevelopment, reduced IQ, impaired psychomotor development, reduced mental and motor skills and even ADHD[1, 5, 8–14].

And while it takes severe deficiency to produce these more conspicuous disorders, mild to moderate deficiency – as seen in Europe and the USA – could have subtle adverse effects. The implications are clear – fall short of iodine in pregnancy and the mental development of your children could be hindered[5, 15].

The mother takes a hit, too. Lack of iodine in pregnancy places a great stress on the mother's thyroid gland, causing functional and anatomical changes. In countries with moderately deficient iodine intakes (such as Ireland, Germany, Belgium, Italy and Denmark), increases in thyroid gland size of 14–30% are observed during pregnancy. This doesn't occur in populations that are iodine sufficient (for example, Finland and the Netherlands)[16].

> **i** It's very important to raise iodine status and ensure good iodine stores in the thyroid *before* pregnancy; taking an iodine supplement after pregnancy has started could actually have an adverse effect.

It's abundantly clear that building up iodine stores before pregnancy, and ensuring an appropriate iodine intake throughout pregnancy and lactation, is a massive priority. While this can be done through diet, for most women a supplement which contains about 150mcg of iodine is the most practical recommendation. In reality, though, that might be easier said than done. Many supplements marketed as suitable for pregnant women don't actually contain iodine, and although 77% of pregnant women will take some form of dietary supplement, only 20% contain supplementary iodine[17]. Ironically, iodine is found in over double the number of supplements consumed by the non-pregnant population![17]. In Europe, only between 13 and 50% of pregnant women (depending on the country) consume prenatal iodine supplements[16].

> **i** Ensure the iodine in your supplement is in the form of potassium iodide. Steer clear of all kelp products. The iodine content of a kelp product might be stated on the label, but what the manufacturer says generally can't be trusted. One study showed that actual iodine amounts ranged from 45–914% of the manufacturer's stated amount[16].

> **i** The richest sources of iodine in our diet are found in fish, seafood, milk, dairy and eggs. The lowest levels are found in plants. The main source of iodine in the UK diet is milk (which makes up 40%) and dairy products, so women who do not consume milk are at special risk of deficiency unless they are big fish or seafood eaters.

> **i** In the UK, organic milk is 42% lower in iodine than conventional milk[18]. As milk is the main source of iodine in the UK, British women who opt for organic milk could be compromising their iodine status.

Vegetarians and vegans need to be especially conscious of the importance of iodine supplementation. Lack of fish and milk can greatly diminish iodine intake[19–21]. In a study of British vegans, it was found that 63% of women had iodine intakes of less than 70mcg per day[22], which is appallingly low. A lot of plant foods that might be especially abundant in vegetarian diets can be 'goitrogenic', impeding iodine utilization and thyroid hormone production. Common examples include cassava, sweet potatoes, the brassicas (cabbage, kale, cauliflower, broccoli and turnip), soy and millet. Some vegans rely on seaweed for their iodine, and while it is an abundant source, it has a massive variation in iodine content and can unwittingly lead to excessive iodine intakes[23], which can also be harmful to the thyroid. For that reason, we don't recommend it. With all this in mind, and to err on the side of caution, vegetarian women should aim for an iodine supplement of up to 200mcg per day before and during pregnancy and lactation, while vegans may need as much as the full 250mcg per day.

> **i** Cigarette smoking produces thiocyanate, which is a goitrogen and reduces iodine uptake by the thyroid. Yet another reason to give up smoking.

Selenium

As we discussed in Chapter 4, while Americans fare well in the selenium stakes, Europe is languishing far behind. The growing foetus needs selenium, and sufficient levels are also needed to reduce the risks of birth complications. Women with lower selenium levels have greater miscarriage rates[24, 25] (miscarriage occurs in 10–20% of pregnancies[26]). Lower selenium levels have been associated with a 440% increased risk of pre-eclampsia[27] (pre-eclampsia occurs in about 3% of pregnancies and causes 60,000 maternal deaths a year[26]). There are also indications that low selenium levels increase the risk of preterm labour[26]. In a study of 1,129 Dutch women who were followed through pregnancy, those with the lowest levels of selenium had twice the risk of preterm birth[28]. In women pregnant for the first time, supplementation with 100mcg of selenium per day reduced premature (pre-labour) rupture of membranes by over 60%[29]. Higher selenium levels may also reduce gestational diabetes risk[26].

We've something important to add to this catalogue of benefits. Selenium is also needed for healthy thyroid function. Low selenium increases oxidative stress and damage to the thyroid[30]. So what do we have in the UK – a double whammy of selenium and iodine deficiency – which means the thyroid takes a real battering during pregnancy, exacerbating the risk of the developing baby being exposed to low thyroid hormone levels, with all the problems that entails, and increasing the risk of the mother developing thyroid problems after birth.

So, as we trumpeted in Chapter 4, it's time for the UK (and Europe) to raise its game and ensure that pregnant women get their fill of selenium by supplementing with 50–60mcg per day.

Vitamin D

We covered vitamin D and its multitude of health benefits earlier in the book. Now we hone in on its role in the precious nine months of pregnancy, and in early life. As you might guess, a low vitamin D level in pregnancy sparks problems. Having a vitamin D level less than 15ng/ml is associated with an almost fivefold increase in the occurrence of pre-eclampsia[31], although not all studies have confirmed this link. In contrast, a higher vitamin D intake during pregnancy is associated with increased birth weight[32], which is highly desirable as a positive predictor of future health. Supplementing with vitamin D as laid out in Chapter 7 for all winter/spring pregnancies will ensure that the mother is vitamin D replete and able to reap these benefits.

Post-birth is when things start to get more complicated. When it comes to the health of the baby and mother alike, breastfeeding is *the* way to go. Despite the almost infinite list of benefits we could cite, breast milk has one tiny flaw – its vitamin D content is extremely poor. And that's the case even if the mother is vitamin D replete. In mothers with high vitamin D levels (32–33ng/ml), the breast milk still contained far too little vitamin D to keep their children sufficient in it[33, 34]. Even mothers supplementing as high as 2,000IU per day was inadequate to supply sufficient vitamin D to the infant[35]. It appears that giving breastfeeding mothers vitamin D supplements of 4,000IU per day is necessary to get enough vitamin D into the infant[36].

Considering that doses of this magnitude are not generally advised for adult use, the solution is to supplement the infant instead. Recommendations from the US Institute of Medicine and American Academy of Pediatrics are for a daily vitamin D intake of 400IU for all infants, beginning in the first few days of life[37]. These recommendations come on the back of research showing that while rickets is typically associated with very low vitamin D levels (<10–11ng/ml), having vitamin D levels as high as 20ng/ml can still cause rickets in some cases[38]. This is a level that the majority of breastfed infants will have without supplementation.

Giving 400IU vitamin D to infants consistently raises levels above 20ng/ml and can even exceed the upper range we recommend for adults (32ng/ml) [34, 37–41]. In Germany, breastfed infants born with sufficient vitamin D levels (27ng/ml) given just 250IU per day saw their levels rise to a massive 55ng/ml after six weeks (the infants also received small amounts of sun exposure)[41]. In a pilot study of children born to mothers at the top end of vitamin D sufficiency (32ng/ml), breastfeeding alone was an inadequate source of vitamin D, but adding a 300IU per day supplement ensured levels were at the top end of sufficiency at month four[34].

Maybe then, the recommendation to give an infant 400IU per day is a bit too generous? We should point out that this recommended intake has a few caveats. First, that infants younger than six months are kept out of the sun altogether, and those aged six months or older wear protective clothing and sunscreen to minimize sun exposure[42]. Second, it is common for infants not to receive the supplement every day (the rate of non-compliance with vitamin D supplements is as high as 45%[41]). Finally, many infants are born to vitamin D deficient mothers and need larger amounts initially.

So for many, to whom these caveats are not applicable, the UK recommendation for supplements of just 280–300IU per day[43] will be more suitable. Alas, the UK only recommends supplementation from six months. For reasons unbeknown to us, they deem breast milk to provide a sufficient supply before this point. As we've seen, though, supplementation is actually necessary from the first few days after birth.

We back the 'breast is best' brigade 100%, but don't be fooled into thinking that breast milk is perfect. Unfortunately, parents don't believe there's a need to supplement their newborns – a survey found that only 16% of breastfed infants received vitamin D supplements[44]. But as we've seen, it was never intended for vitamin D to come from the diet, and since we vigorously protect our children from the sun, supplementation is a necessity.

Infant formulas are fortified with vitamin D. Once formula-fed infants are ingesting sufficient formula to achieve a vitamin D intake of 300–400IU per day, they will be receiving an adequate intake and will not require supplementation.

Iron

If there's one thing that gets drummed into pregnant women, it's that they need iron. It's no wonder, when we consider that iron deficiency is rife, occurring in up to 40% of pregnant women in the West[45]. And that's certainly not a good thing, with iron deficiency in pregnancy associated with a greater than twofold increase in the risk of preterm delivery[46]. What's more, it increases the risk of a low birth weight and can impair intelligence and motor and behavioural development in the child[45]. In studies of iron-replete women, iron supplements (30mg per day) gave rise to children with a higher birth weight[47] and reduced preterm deliveries[48].

So getting your fill of iron in pregnancy is clearly a good thing. The hitch, once again, is that our typical intakes are pretty poor. Figures from the 2001 National Diet and Nutrition Survey in the UK showed an average intake of 10mg for women aged 19–64 (well below the recommended daily intake of 15mg)[3]. In the USA, only about a quarter of females aged 12–49 hit the 15mg mark[49]. The upshot is that a lot of women enter pregnancy with low iron reserves, or worse still, already iron deficient[50]. Pregnancy adds further to the demand for iron, meaning that as pregnancy progresses, the prevalence of iron deficiency increases. Data from the NHANES study in the USA showed that, while 7% of pregnant women were iron deficient in the first trimester, this increased to 30% by the third trimester[51]. In the first trimester, the increased requirements are easily met by the savings made by not menstruating. However, needs rise in the second trimester to between 4–5mg per day[52] (normal requirements are 1–2mg per day), and in the third trimester to 6mg or more per day, as iron accumulation in the foetus really picks up pace. For the last six to eight weeks the need for iron can be as much as 10mg per day[52].

That doesn't sound too bad though, right? Even with poor intakes surely we're easily hitting the 6mg per day mark? The big snag with iron is that it's poorly absorbed, and the typical 10mg intake seen in the UK diet won't even come close. Even with the body increasing its ability to absorb iron as pregnancy progresses, the best-case scenario is for 30% of the iron from the diet to be absorbed[53]. So, even with a diet rich in highly bioavailable iron, women still fall short of meeting their iron needs, hitting only about 1.9mg in the second trimester and 5mg in the third[52].

And that only really leaves one solution: to supplement iron in order to prevent deficiency. Guidelines vary considerably. The World Health Organization (WHO) recommends 60mg per day for six months during pregnancy, and even to increase the amount to 120mg if it is to be taken for less than six months[45]. The US Center for Disease Control recommends a 'low-dose' 30mg iron supplement during pregnancy, as well as a diet high in iron and vitamin C to aid its absorption[49]. And the UK? True to form, the UK doesn't recommend universal supplementation. It maintains that the recommended daily intake of 15mg is enough, advising that pregnant women should have sufficient stores coming into pregnancy and that increased absorption from the diet will cover it[53].

Although the UK appears to lag behind the USA in nutrition, first with selenium, and then with vitamin D, in the case of iron it comes up trumps. We've focused on the benefits of iron in pregnancy so far, but that all-too-familiar 'more is better' mentality rears its ugly head again. Correcting iron deficiency is one thing, but universal supplementation is quite another, and takes us into questionable territory[46]. The wisdom of this approach has been questioned by a Cochrane Review, which found insufficient evidence that blanket treatment in pregnancy improves functional and health outcomes for women and babies[54].

It's one thing to find no benefit, but quite another to discover that it may even cause harm. And that's exactly what is happening. When it comes to iron, a delicate balance is needed. Get too gung ho with it and you run into problems. High iron levels are now linked to the development of gestational diabetes and pre-eclampsia, as well as increased oxidative stress[46, 55]. It has also been suggested that building up the mother's iron stores will increase the thickness of the blood, hindering placental blood flow to the uterus[46]. Besides, we shouldn't forget that high iron intakes can interfere with the intestinal absorption of other essential nutrients (e.g. zinc, copper, chromium, molybdenum, manganese, magnesium and calcium), many of which have important roles[53]. Iron supplements also have side effects, especially at high doses, such as stomach upset, nausea, diarrhoea and constipation – pregnancy is good enough at causing these problems without getting outside help.

Despite all of these concerns, a study in the USA found that about 70% of pregnant and lactating women were taking iron supplements, the mid-range dose being 60mg per day. Yet less than 15% of women of reproductive age taking iron supplements had reason to believe they were at risk of anaemia[46]. It is naïve to think that blanket supplementation carries no risks for those who have no need for extra iron. That's why the National Institute of Clinical Excellence (NICE) in the UK only advocates supplements after low haemoglobin levels have been measured. This seems to make more sense as it identifies exactly which pregnant women require iron supplementation. While NICE recommends the measurement of haemoglobin levels, we must warn that such an approach has been found to be insensitive and that a measure of iron stores (ferritin) should be taken as well. Iron sufficiency is indicated by a haemoglobin level greater than 110g/L and a serum ferritin of 12mcg/L or greater in early pregnancy[56].

> **i** The amount of iron we absorb from a supplement reduces as the dose increases. The absorption rate of a 5mg dose of iron is about 36% towards the end of pregnancy but only 14% from a 100mg dose[52].

> **i** Consuming tea or coffee with, or shortly after, a meal dramatically inhibits the absorption of dietary iron. In contrast, vitamin C-rich foods greatly enhance absorption.

> **i** Foods rich in iron include meats (especially red meat), beans, tofu, nuts, most dark green leafy vegetables (e.g. kale and watercress) and dried fruits such as dried apricots.

DHA

Docosahexaenoic acid, or DHA for short, is the predominant omega-3 fat found in the retina of the eye and the central nervous system, making it of great importance for foetal growth, and especially brain development[57]. It accumulates rapidly in the brain, particularly in the last trimester, when development really takes off, with the brain amassing a staggering 67mg per day[58]. You'd be right in thinking this is a pretty important type of fat in any pregnancy, and evidence has grown to suggest that insufficient intakes of DHA can have a range of unwanted consequences, including increased postnatal depression, preterm and low weight births and pre-eclampsia[58].

An insufficient supply of DHA to the infant during pregnancy may result in permanent impairment of learning ability[59]. Visual acuity may be hampered and immune system development blunted increasing the occurrence of allergies[58]. But where exactly does the DHA come from for all this important stuff to happen? The maternal diet – which means that DHA availability throughout pregnancy, and breastfeeding, is dependent on the mother's dietary intake[57].

And herein lies the problem. Several expert groups recommend average DHA intakes of 200–300mg per day to meet the needs of pregnancy[60]. That's all well and good, but the Western diet falls way, way short of this, providing a paltry 60–80mg daily[60]. Hitting the recommended two servings of fish a week (one of them oily fish) would give a sufficient DHA intake, but just 19% of Americans meet this recommendation[61]. With the recent scares about contaminants in fish (such as mercury and polychlorinated biphenyls), many people have reduced their fish intake, a drop seen most noticeably in pregnant women[60].

And what a shame! Compared with mothers who consume more than 340g of seafood per week, mothers who consume no seafood have a 48% increased risk of their children being in the lowest quartile for verbal IQ[62]. A low maternal intake of seafood was also linked with a greater risk of poorer developmental outcomes on a range of behaviour, fine motor, communication and social development scores[62]. While it's not possible to say exactly which component of seafood was having this positive effect – for example, it could have been due to the iodine rather than omega-3 – it does provide proof of principle that, when it comes to fish, the benefits of eating it far outweigh the risks of avoiding it. This is supported by the FDA and the Institute of Medicine, both of which concur that the benefits of consuming fish during pregnancy outweigh the risks[60]. Avoiding tilefish, swordfish, shark, and king mackerel, and limiting albacore tuna to no more than 170g per week, is recommended. For those who still wish to shy away from fish, the alternative is a DHA supplement. With the purity of these also questionable, it's essential to ensure you go for a brand that guarantees quality and is produced to 'good manufacturing practices'.

> **i** Just 170g of Atlantic salmon provides over 2,400mg of DHA. Choosing wild over farmed varieties and trimming away the fatty areas before cooking will reduce PCB intake[60].

> **i** Being vegetarian or vegan doesn't mean you have to scrimp on your DHA intake, as supplements derived from algae offer an excellent vegetarian source of DHA.

Folic acid

Last, but by no means least, the one we've all heard of: folic acid. Neural tube defects are among the most common types of birth defect[63], with spina bifida and anencephaly, caused by the incomplete closing of the spine and skull, occurring in about three in every 10,000 live births[64]. This equates to about 3,000 cases in the USA each year[65]. It is now well established that a diet high in folate reduces this risk dramatically. Folate is found in high amounts in the likes of green leafy vegetables, broccoli, Brussels sprouts, asparagus, peas, chickpeas, citrus fruits and brown rice. However, only about half of the folate in the diet is absorbed, and cooking practices – such as stewing, processing and storage – can also reduce folate content. This means that, without care, diet alone can be insufficient to supply the necessary amounts of folate needed by prospective mothers. For this reason, massive campaigns have been undertaken to promote supplementation of folic acid before conception and in the first trimester of pregnancy. Folic acid is a synthetic derivative of folate with a greater stability and superior absorption. Taking just 400mcg per day before and during pregnancy could prevent up to 70% of neural tube defects[65].

> **i** It has also been proposed that folic acid may reduce preterm birth, pre-eclampsia, placental abruption, intrauterine growth restriction and foetal death[63]. However, the evidence is just suggestive and nowhere near the strength of evidence that exists for neural tube defect prevention.

Alas, despite all the education and publicity, folate levels in pregnancy remained low, with 25% of US women still folate deficient during pregnancy[63]. In the UK, it's estimated that over 13 million people currently consume too little folic acid in their diet[66]. In response, compulsory fortification of products like flour, rice, pasta, bread and cereals with folic acid was introduced in the USA in 1998. By 2008, 52 countries had instituted fortification programmes and their success is believed to have reduced the prevalence of neural tube defects by an impressive 46%[63].

However, mandatory folic acid fortification was not introduced in the UK. After careful consideration, the UK opted out, based on concerns that giving high amounts to the non-pregnant population could cause unforeseen problems. For instance, high levels could mask a vitamin B12 deficiency, facilitate the progression of early cancer formations and hinder the activity of anti-folate medications used in rheumatoid arthritis and cancer[63, 67].

Irrespective of fortification programmes, it is recommended that all women trying to conceive supplement 400mcg per day of folic acid, or consume a product with a known 400mcg content, such as many cereals in the USA[66]. And here's the important bit. Folic acid works its magic in the first 28 days after conception, before the closure of the neural tube. This makes it crucial for women to start supplementing one month before conception and throughout the first trimester. Considering that half of all pregnancies are unplanned[65], all women of childbearing age should routinely supplement with folic acid. Yet, despite all the education campaigns, only 12% of women are aware of this fact[65].

If you are obese, you run a particularly high risk of being deficient in folate. In 2010, the UK *Guidelines for Management of Women with Obesity in Pregnancy* recommended the folic acid dose be upped to 5mg in women with a BMI over 30, one month before conception and for the first trimester[66]. Women with diabetes and epilepsy are also at considerable risk and should follow this advice for increased intakes[66].

THE PARTING SHOT

The health and wellbeing of our children is without question a most precious thing. Given the choice, it's not something that any parent is going to compromise. Following standard advice for healthy eating in pregnancy is undoubtedly a good start. But why settle for second best?

It is patently obvious that simply eating a 'well-balanced diet' is just not enough. Stick with that idea and there's every chance that critical vitamins, minerals and omega-3 fats will fall short of the mark. But supplying the mother with all the pieces of the nutritional jigsaw before, during and after pregnancy (ensuring neither too much, nor too little), not only minimizes the risk of complications but sets the stage for a bright and prosperous future that will allow future generations to flourish.

SUMMARY AND RECOMMENDATIONS

- Iodine is critically important for a baby's mental development and supplements of about 150mcg per day should be started preconceptionally and continued throughout pregnancy and lactation. Vegetarians, and especially vegans, may need 200–250mcg per day.

- For selenium-depleted populations such as the UK (see Chapter 4) a supplement of 50–60mcg per day should be taken.

- Mothers should ensure their vitamin D levels are adequately topped up (see Chapter 7). From the first days after birth, breastfed infants and those not consuming 300–400IU a day from formula, should be supplemented with vitamin D daily.

- Iron deficiency in pregnancy is prevalent, but this does not justify universal high-dose supplementation. Insist your doctor measures your haemoglobin and ferritin levels before any iron supplementation regime is commenced.

- Women who eat little or no fish should take a supplement providing 200–300mg of DHA during pregnancy and breastfeeding. Vegetarians and vegans can take DHA supplements derived from algae. When buying formula for infants, ensure DHA is a listed ingredient.

- Folic acid supplements of 400mcg per day should be taken by all women of childbearing age, and continued for the first trimester of pregnancy. For the obese, diabetics and epileptics, a dose of 5mg is advised for one month prior to conception and throughout the first trimester, under medical supervision.

PART VI
FAILING FATS

'Any man can make mistakes, but only
an idiot persists in his error.'
MARCUS TULLIUS CICERO, LAWYER, AUTHOR,
SCHOLAR, ORATOR AND STATESMAN (106–43BC)

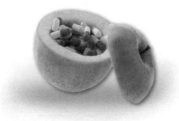

CHAPTER 16
A BIG FAT MISTAKE

OVERVIEW

- Could one of our most prominent public health messages – to cut down on saturated fat – be fundamentally flawed?
- Worse still, could what we replace it with in our diets be doing even more damage?
- We challenge the orthodox view that simply eating more carbs, or more polyunsaturated fats, is the way to go.
- Forget saturated fats – the real answer to our heart health woes lie elsewhere.

If there's one thing we know when it comes to heart disease prevention, it's the need to reduce our intake of saturated fat. This is one of the pillars of international dietary health recommendations. And the message must have got through. A mighty 73% of Americans now know that saturated fat can cause heart disease[1]; 61% of the UK 'correctly' know we should be eating less saturated fat[2]. The UK's Food Standards Agency states that a small drop in saturated fat intake (from 13.3% of calories to 11% or less) would save 3,500 lives a year, not to mention £1 billion for the economy[3].

The evidence for saturated fat and heart disease sure looks conclusive. Because here's the thing: saturated fat raises your 'bad' LDL cholesterol, which is a cast-iron cause of heart disease[4].

> **i** The top five dietary sources of saturated fat in the UK are dairy (24%), meat (22%), fat spreads (11%), biscuits (cookies) and baked goods (8%), and chocolate confectionary (5%).

A sugar-coated fiasco

We can replace saturated fat with any nutrient – protein, carbohydrate, monounsaturated fats or polyunsaturated fats – and our LDL cholesterol levels reduce[5, 6]. And with it goes our risk of heart disease... or so we've been told. The truth is, we've made a big fat mess out of it all. The way the unrelenting message is drummed into us, you'd think the evidence was watertight, wouldn't you? Actually, it's non-existent!

It may sound like heresy, but the research is there to back it. In 2010, a meta-analysis of 21 studies encompassing 347,747 subjects found no evidence to conclude that dietary saturated fat was associated with an increased risk of coronary heart disease, stroke or cardiovascular disease[7]. We know, that bit of information got our eyebrows raised, too.

> **i** Considering that negative studies are less likely to be published, and the low number of published studies on saturated fat that exist compared to the international attention it has received, we have to wonder how many other studies exonerating saturated fat have not made it into the public domain.

A large Japanese cohort study, also published in 2010, following 58,453 men and women for 14 years, found that those who consumed between 2.5g–11g of saturated fat per day (so, what would be deemed 'ideal') had a staggering 45% increased risk of stroke compared to those eating 18g or more per day, as well as a 22% increase in the risk of cardiovascular disease[8]. So where is all this compelling evidence that has tainted the reputation of saturated fats?

Irrespective of the lack of hard evidence over the last few decades, the 'fat is bad' mantra has hit home. Total fat and saturated fat intake has declined. And if something goes down in our diet, then something else will go up. As we've been banishing the fats, we've made up for them with a compensatory increase in carbohydrate intake. Data from the USA shows that about 50% of our calories now come from carbohydrates[9]. High-carb, low-fat diets rule, and when it comes to heart disease, this should be a good thing, right?

For every 1% increase in energy intake from saturated fat in place of carbohydrates, our 'bad' LDL cholesterol increases by about 0.03mmol/L[10]. All sounds good, in theory, but what about in reality? An analysis of US and European cohort studies found that if we replace just 5% of our energy intake from saturated fats with carbohydrates (such a drop would put us at recommended levels), we see a 7% increase in coronary events[11]. The thing is, when it comes to heart disease and cholesterol, it's not just about our LDL levels. To look only at this factor, and ignore everything else, is far too simplistic. Carbohydrates can increase triglycerides[12] (which are an established risk factor for heart disease) and decrease the 'good' HDL cholesterol[12].

But it doesn't stop there, and we need to go back to LDL. Sure, switch your saturated fats to carbs and your amount of LDL decreases, but what we're rarely told is that not all LDL is the same; it can differ by its particle size. And anything that increases triglyceride levels, such as carbs, increases the amount of what's known as 'small low density LDL'[13, 14]. It appears that these small LDL particles have a much greater atherogenicity – meaning they'll clog up your artery walls in no time. Their smaller size allows greater penetration into the artery walls, reduces their ability to bind to the LDL receptor, which causes them to stay in our bloodstream longer, and makes them more susceptible to oxidation. It appears these negative effects of high carbohydrate intake are especially pronounced in the overweight population, which unfortunately is now the majority [12].

When it comes to carbohydrates and risk of heart disease, it's all about the quality of carbohydrate, which can be measured by its Glycemic Index (GI) – in other words, how high our blood sugar levels rise after consumption. In a cohort study of 53,644 men and women over 12 years, it was the high GI foods (the refined carbohydrates) which had a devastating effect on heart health [15]. Replacing 5% of calories from saturated fat with high-glycemic carbs was associated with a whopping 33% increase in heart attack occurrence. Switching saturated fat for medium GI carbs had no effect, whereas there was a suggestion that low GI carbs could possibly even lower the risk. It's not hard to see how low GI carbohydrates wouldn't increase risk, and may be beneficial. Here we're talking about minimally processed grains, legumes, fruit and vegetables. So with these foods, we're not just talking carbohydrates, but vitamins, minerals, phytonutrients and fibre, all of which are essential for overall and cardiovascular health. As well as this, it seems the deleterious effects of these 'good' carbohydrates on our lipid profile might be minimal [12].

That's all well and good, but this pattern of eating hardly defines the Western diet, does it? Our penchant is for high GI carbohydrates, which are all too often stripped of nutrients. We're talking about the highly processed beige and white foods – bread and other baked goods, rice, pasta, breakfast cereals, potatoes and beverages – that characterize the Western diet. Not to mention the multitude of cleverly marketed goods lining our shelves that are laden with added sugar (they are supposedly 'okay' because they are 'low fat' – what a joke). What we're left with is a continual sugar dump into our bloodstream, and the accompanying hormonal chaos that ensues, which leads to oxidative stress, inflammation, beta cell dysfunction and endothelial dysfunction[16]. Add to this raised triglycerides, reduced HDL and smaller LDL particle size, and it's not difficult to see how high-GI junk dramatically increases our risk of heart disease.

To us, it's become apparent that the hallowed public health message to reduce saturated fat, so loudly trumpeted, has backfired. It is a travesty and detrimental to our cardiovascular health. In the words of one researcher, 'the obesity epidemic and growing intake of refined carbohydrates have created a "perfect storm" for the development of cardio-metabolic disorders'[17].

Stolen credit

So, recommendations are now to replace saturated fat with polyunsaturated fats (or 'PUFAs' for short). Whereas saturated fats are mainly hard animal fats, polyunsaturated fats are mainly liquid vegetable oils. In a review of eight RCTs totalling 13,614 participants, it was found that if we switch 5% of our calorie intake from saturated fats to polyunsaturated fats, our coronary heart disease risk reduces by an impressive 10%[18]. A meta-analysis of 60 trials found replacing carbohydrates with polyunsaturated fats had the most favourable effect on improving our cholesterol profiles[10].

There are two main types of polyunsaturated fats – omega-3 and omega-6. But with the omega-3s present in few food sources and only needed in relatively small amounts, they don't offer an appropriate substitute for our saturated fat intake. Thus it is the omega-6s, with their much greater availability and consumption levels, that have received the accolades[19]. But that doesn't mean that our heart disease woes are over. The fact is that government health agencies around the world have set a recommended limit on omega-6 consumption, which is typically an intake of about 4–8% of energy[19, 20]. The US National Cholesterol Education Program states that 'there are no large populations that have consumed large quantities of polyunsaturated fatty acids for long periods. Thus, high intakes have not been proven safe in large populations; this introduces a note of caution for recommending high intakes'[21].

> **i** Omega-6 fats are found in vegetable oils – such as sunflower, corn, soybean, safflower and sesame – margarines, nuts, seeds, cereal grains and many processed foods (in the form of linoleic acid), and in meats, poultry, eggs and dairy products (in the form of arachidonic acid).

The big worry is that, on a biochemical level, eating too much omega-6 could contribute to inflammation in the body because the main type of omega-6 in the diet, linoleic acid, can be converted into arachidonic acid, which the body can then utilize to make pro-inflammatory chemicals[19]. While many people, including scientists, are concerned by this factor, it doesn't actually appear to happen in humans because the conversion process is tightly regulated. So, even with higher intakes of linoleic acid, the increased conversion to arachidonic acid is minimal[22]. And contrary to what many think, it seems that a high omega-6 intake could even bring about a reduced inflammatory state[19, 23]. But it is still all rather ambiguous and recommendations for upper intakes of omega-6 remain in place (with the exception of The American Heart Association, which recommends a minimum 5–10% of energy intake from omega-6 fats[19]).

So where does that leave us? Well, the omega-6 linoleic acid already makes up over 7% of energy intake in our diet[24]. This is predominantly through the greater than 1000-fold increase in soybean oil consumption that occurred in the twentieth century[24]. So what's the point in recommending that we replace saturated fats with yet more omega-6 when we're already consuming towards the upper end of recommended levels anyway? Considering that our alarming rates of heart disease have been accompanied by a dramatic rise in omega-6 consumption, are we really sure this is the table upon which we want to lay our bets?

One researcher who was unhappy to do so was Christopher Ramsden. When it comes to the trials that hail the polyunsaturated fats, we're essentially talking about vegetable oils. While they are made up mostly of omega-6s, they also contain some omega-3s, which is worth mentioning. Ramsden and his colleagues, suspicious of the accolades accorded to the omega-6s, took the trials that were included in the meta-analyses for polyunsaturated fats and coronary heart disease risk and did something very interesting[25]. They split the trials into those that just increased omega-6 and those which used a mixed intervention increasing both omega-3s and omega-6s. The results were sobering indeed. RCTs that replaced saturated fat with just omega-6s produced no reduction in coronary heart disease. If anything, there were suggestions of an increased risk! So there we have it: another nutrient purported to save us from those 'noxious' saturated fats that just doesn't hold up when put under scrutiny.

Unsung hero

With this revelation we see that it's not the omega-6s that should be adorned with all the plaudits, but the omega-3s. More specifically, it's the omega-3 fats EPA and DHA – the ones we find in oily fish – that are the true champions of our cardiovascular health. And are we so surprised? Just under 1g of EPA/DHA per day in a post-heart attack population is clinically proven to reduce death, non-fatal heart attack and non-fatal stroke by about 15%[26]. Omega-3s assist in stabilizing the electrical activity of the heart and in so doing, reduce the chances of developing arrhythmias, or an abnormal heart rhythmn[27]. Omega-3s are anti-thrombogenic (reducing the risk of blood clots), anti-inflammatory and therefore anti-atherogenic, and to top it off even have small effects on lowering blood pressure[27].

Omega-3s lower triglyceride levels, with higher amounts used as an extremely effective treatment for hypertriglyceridemia, and thus decrease our small density LDL amounts, too. The omega-3 intake of the Japanese, with their fish-rich diet, hits near a gram per day, and they have extremely low levels of heart disease[28]. Here in the West, recommendations are to eat two servings of fish per week, of which one should be oily fish, and while even this may be a bit on the low side, only 19% of us achieve it[29]. As a result, our omega-3 EPA and DHA intake is a paltry 100–200mg per day[30]. Unsurprisingly, heart disease is rampant.

> **i** Amounts of fish supplying a gram of EPA/DHA are: herring 42–56g; salmon (farmed) 42–70g, (wild) 56–98g; trout (85–98g); mackerel 56–238g; shrimp 308g; tuna (drained light tinned) 336g; cod (Atlantic) 350g, (Pacific) 644g; and haddock 420g[31].

> **i** The beneficial health effects of omega-3 fish oils were first described in the Greenland Inuit. Consuming a diet rich in seafood appeared to proffer significant protection against coronary heart disease.

When we talk about omega-3, we're essentially talking about fish, because no other dietary source comes close. In a 30-year trial of men (aged 40–55) in Chicago, eating an average of 35g of fish a day meant you had a 38% lower risk of death from coronary heart disease compared to those who didn't eat fish[32]. A meta-analysis of 19 observational studies found that fish consumption was associated with a 14% lower risk of total coronary heart disease occurrence compared with little or no fish consumption[33].

Omega-3 fats in the form of alpha-linolenic acid are found in some vegetable oils (e.g. rapeseed/canola and flax), some nuts and seeds (e.g. walnut and flax) and green leafy vegetables. However, the more potent forms of EPA and DHA omega-3 are found in cold-water fish and seafood.

Experts agree that we need a minimum of 500mg per day of EPA plus DHA combined to maintain cardiovascular health[34]. Consuming this level would be expected to significantly reduce the risk of death from coronary heart disease in healthy adults. For those with coronary heart disease, intakes of 1g per day are advised[31].

Heart health is really only the beginning of the omega-3 story, and to stop there would do it an injustice. While the omega-6 fat arachidonic acid gets converted into pro-inflammatory factors in the body, the omega-3s fight aggressively for these same pathways to produce their less inflammatory factors. The upshot is that the omega-3-generated ones dampen down the overall inflammatory response. Getting sufficient omega-3 means that we can curb the activity of arachidonic acid in the body and with it reduce our levels of inflammation. Without sufficient omega-3 to keep arachidonic acid in check, we begin to see just why inflammation can become rampant in anyone following a typical Western diet. And that's something to be wary of, as evidence is gathering to suggest that inflammation has a role to play in such diverse conditions as neurodegenerative diseases, obesity, type 2 diabetes, even cancer, to name but a few [35, 36]. When it comes to the classic inflammatory disease, rheumatoid arthritis, data consistently shows an improvement in symptoms from using fish oils, although a minimum intake of 3g per day of EPA plus DHA combined is required for effective results[37, 38].

Fish stocks in the sea are under threat, so buy fish from sustainable sources wherever possible.

Now we must turn our attention to vegetarians and vegans. As we've seen in previous chapters, their predominant source of omega-3 is through plants providing alpha linolenic acid. And the conversion of this to the more potent EPA and DHA is poor. For these groups, their omega-6 to omega-3 ratio is of the utmost importance; ideally they should be striving for 4:1 or less. To achieve this they need to limit omega-6 oils. This can be done by switching from oils to wholefood sources such as sunflower seeds, pumpkin seeds, sesame seeds, walnuts, wheat germ and soy foods[39]. These provide smaller overall amounts of omega-6, while contributing other vital nutrients. Likewise, placing a greater emphasis on the omega-9 monounsaturated fats found in nuts, olives and olive oil, avocados and rapeseed/canola oil is a good strategy.

> **i** Little attention is given to monounsaturated fatty acids, but we could all probably benefit from increasing them. Monounsaturated-rich olive oil is a core component of the Mediterranean diet, which is strongly linked with lower cardiovascular and other inflammatory diseases[40].

Incorporating good sources of the plant form of omega-3, alpha linolenic acid, is a must – good sources of this include flaxseed, hempseed, rapeseed/canola, walnuts and legumes (soy), as well as green leafy vegetables. A supplement of DHA-enriched microalgae (up to 300mg per day) is also encouraged[39]. DHA can also be converted back to EPA in small amounts in the body, helping to raise our EPA levels this way[45].

> **i** Prime examples of omega-6-laden oils include safflower oil (75% omega-6), grapeseed oil (70% omega-6), sunflower oil (65% omega-6), corn oil (57% omega-6), cottonseed oil (52% omega-6), and soybean oil (51% omega-6)[39].

THE SCIENCE BLAST: OMEGA OILS

So, there's a bit of a competition going on here between omega-3 and omega-6, and it's an idea that has fuelled the notion that we should aim to consume an 'ideal' ratio of these fats in our diet. If we look back to our hunter-gatherer ancestors, their natural diet would have provided a ratio of omega-6 to omega-3 fats of about 1–2:1[41]. Just compare that to the ratio in our modern Western diet, which is more like 10:1[24] and could even be as high as 30:1![41] Because omega-6 can compete for the same enzymes and pathways in the body as omega-3, it's proposed that scoffing large amounts of omega-6 (exactly as we see today) will overwhelm our omega-3, cancelling out their anti-inflammatory benefits.

However, most of our intake of omega-6 comes in the form of linoleic acid and, as we've seen, its conversion to arachidonic acid is tightly controlled, meaning that even the high amounts we consume are having a negligible impact. And while linoleic acid can compete with the omega-3s for incorporation into tissues, it seems it can also kick out arachidonic acid, so the net effect may actually be an anti-inflammatory one[24]. In the Los Angeles Veterans Study, a diet high in linoleic acid (15% of energy) actually reduced the amount of arachidonic acid in coronary atheroma phospholipids by 40%[42]. A US study found that, not only did linoleic acid intake not impede the anti-inflammatory actions of omega-3, but the greatest anti-inflammatory effect was seen from a combination of both omega-6 and omega-3[43]. So you might hear a lot of talk about getting the correct ratio of omega-6 to omega-3, but you can forget it. It's not the ratio that matters, it's about bumping up our omega-3 intake to a meaningful level to reap the beneficial effects.

There is one caveat if you are a vegetarian or a vegan. Up to now when we've talked about omega-3, it's been pretty much synonymous with fish. That's because fish provides the potent omega-3 fats EPA and DHA. But plants also provide a type of omega-3 called alpha linolenic acid, which is converted in the body to EPA/DHA. As we know, this conversion process is pretty poor, which means that alpha linolenic acid accounts for quite a negligible supply of EPA/DHA. But what if you don't eat any fish and rely solely on plant sources instead? This is where the omega-6 to omega-3 ratio (or more specifically the linoleic acid to alpha linolenic acid ratio) is crucial.

Linoleic acid actually inhibits the conversion of alpha linolenic acid to EPA and then to DHA[19]. The flipside is that if you reduce linoleic acid and increase alpha linolenic acid it has the effect of reducing conversion to arachidonic acid and increasing conversion to EPA[22, 44]. Therefore, vegetarians should not only increase their intake of omega-3 alpha linolenic acid, but also reduce their omega-6 linoleic acid intake at the same time.

i The enzymes that convert plant omega-3 fatty acids are highly dependent on our nutritional status, requiring adequate levels of pyridoxine, biotin, calcium, copper, magnesium and zinc[39].

i Alcohol inhibits conversion enzymes and depletes tissues of omega-3 fatty acids[39].

THE PARTING SHOT

We've all been part of a big fat experiment, the results of which are out and they're not good. Saturated fat was branded as public health enemy number one and we got so focused on it that we missed the true dietary disaster as our consumption of refined carbohydrates ran amok. So then we switched to the benefits of polyunsaturated fatty acids, and heralded the omega-6s as our saviour. Well, the results are coming back to roost there too, and it's time to question the omega-6 'heart healthy' certificate of authenticity. While not necessarily bad for us, it would be foolhardy to recommend any nutrient whose workings are not fully understood. There's only one solution, and that's to address the elephant in the room.

Saturated fat is simply not deserving of the bad rap it has received. That's not a carte blanche to eat as much of it as you like – if we go to extremes there's likely to be a price to pay. That's the whole point here, getting back to the idea of balance. The reality is, the body is smart and all in all does a pretty good job in maintaining the status quo, as long as we do our bit too. The key is to give the body all the nutrients it needs to do this job, and right now that's being prevented by the staggeringly low intake of omega-3 in our modern diet. If we are to tackle the burden of cardiovascular disease, promoting their intake is the road we have to take.

SUMMARY AND RECOMMENDATIONS

- Strong evidence implicating saturated fat in heart disease doesn't exist.

- If you cut down on saturated fats and replace them with high GI carbohydrates, however, you will dramatically increase your risk of heart disease.

- Replacing saturated fats with omega-6 polyunsaturated fats is a dubious strategy too.

- It's the omega-3 fats EPA and DHA that are truly deserving of our attention and our requirements can be satisfied by consuming two 170g servings of fish a week, with an emphasis on oily fish.

CHAPTER 17
BRAIN DRAIN

OVERVIEW

- Whichever way we look at it, we're faced with a massive burden of mental health problems in the modern world.

- Could our modern-day diet be messing with our brains?

- We explore whether the modern-day epidemics of depression, anti-social behaviour and dementia could be curbed by simple dietary changes?

- In particular, we hone in on fish and its omega-3 fat content, and reveal whether it really is 'brain food'.

We don't hear all that much about mental illness. It is a pretty scary thing after all. When it comes to dinner party etiquette, it's said that of all the subjects to keep quiet about, mental health tops the list, above politics, sex or religion. Despite attempts to increase awareness, we have to admit that mental illness remains a taboo for many of us. You might be forgiven then for not knowing the shocking numbers. Mental illness is a greater health burden in the Western world than any other disease, including cancer and heart disease. Across 30 European countries in a typical year, it's estimated that around 165 million people (we're talking 38% of the total population of these countries) will have a fully developed mental illness[1]. One in four adults in the USA is suffering from a mental illness, and nearly half will develop at least one mental illness in their lifetime[2]. If that's all not too much, let's add in the economic cost of mental illness, which in the USA was $300 billion in 2002, and we can only presume that's got a whole lot worse since[2].

There's no getting away from it: our mental wellbeing in the twenty-first century is in crisis. The burden of brain disorders we now face is unnerving. It's a complex problem, with many different opinions as to how we arrived at this dire state of affairs. But how often do we stop to think that the physical and the mental may not be so disconnected after all, and that the food, and specifically the fats, we eat could be affecting our grey matter?

Depression – not all in the mind

Across 30 European countries, the number of people affected by major depression is a shocking 30 million[1], and around one in ten in the USA are depressed, right now[3]. We've got a serious problem on an epic scale. There are various drugs touted for depression, but they're not much to shout about. Just take the most popular class, selective serotonin reuptake inhibitors (SSRIs for short), where we see a reported 27% discontinuation rate[4] and less than 60% of those who complete a course finding benefit[5]. So it's pretty interesting to see that there's a strong correlation between a nation's fish consumption and the prevalence of depression[6]. In fact, the annual prevalence of major depression shows close to a 60-fold variation across countries[6]. What that means is that countries such as Japan, with a high intake of fish, have the lowest rates of depression, whereas countries with a low intake of fish, like the USA and much of Europe, have the highest. Even within a country, consuming more fish has been shown to correlate with less chance of having depressive symptoms[7].

These might be mere correlations but they make you sit up and listen. Of course, we've got to ask, is it biologically plausible? Well, there can be little doubt that omega-3 fish oils are critical for both the structure and function of the brain, and importantly, they play a role in how our potent brain messengers – neurotransmitters – work[8]. So it does seem feasible that they could affect our mood. Indeed, when researchers have looked at the actual levels of omega-3 fats in depressed patients, they find lower quantities[9], and what's more, the lower the level of omega-3, the worse the depression[10]. Results from studies like these imply that depression is associated with a low intake and/or some sort of abnormal metabolism of omega-3 fats. So, the plot thickens.

Let's up the ante and take a look at the results from more definitive, cut-and-dried, intervention studies. It's not difficult to find studies that show clear benefits from giving supplements of omega-3 fish oils to depressed patients. In a four-week study, giving patients with depression 2g of EPA per day (a specific type of omega-3 fat found in fish oil), alongside their ongoing antidepressant treatment, resulted in significant benefit in depressive symptoms[11]. Another study in patients with persistent depression despite treatment, found that supplementation with 1g per day of EPA resulted in better outcomes on each of the three ratings scales of depression used, compared with those receiving placebos[12]. These encouraging findings from omega-3 fish oil supplements have also been observed in childhood depression[13], as well as depression during pregnancy[14].

The problem is, however, that a bunch of other studies haven't found benefits from fish oil supplements[15–18], so you'd be forgiven for thinking that, overall, the evidence is all a bit shaky. When we have conflicting evidence like this, the best thing to do is to perform a meta-analysis, which basically involves collecting all the relevant studies together and looking for any overall effect. And in September 2011 that's exactly what was done. A meta-analysis of 13 of the relevant and best RCTs of fish oil and major depression was published in the journal *Molecular Psychiatry*[5]. The authors described the results as 'sobering'. While early trials showed much promise, the inclusion of later more rigorously conducted studies showed 'that omega-3 FAs (fatty acids) have, at most, minimal efficacy in treating depression'. So that's apparently that – fish oils are ineffective.

Well, that is if you excuse an oversight. *Molecular Psychiatry* was not the only journal to publish a meta-analysis of fish oils and major depression that month – *The Journal of Clinical Psychiatry* was also in on the act. They examined 15 RCTs (12 of which were the same as the first meta-analysis, so largely the same body of evidence). However, they took a different and more intricate approach to the literature. Building on previous evidence[19], they didn't take fish oils as a whole, instead they examined the individual constituents EPA and DHA. And this time, it gave some very different findings. The thing is, when it comes to fish oils, EPA and DHA are structurally very similar but biologically different. Lump all the studies together and you might easily miss this fact. And here's the thing. It looks likely that it's EPA that's effective in depression, while DHA is not only ineffective, it blocks EPA's activity. And this is exactly what was borne out in the meta-analysis published in *The Journal of Clinical Psychiatry*[20].

The authors found that it was only when EPA was given at levels greater than 60% of the total amount of EPA/DHA that a beneficial effect was observed in depression. As well as this, EPA appears to exert a 'U'-shaped curve, with effects seen only when EPA is in the range of 200–2,200mg greater than DHA. Giving more doesn't do the job. Quite why EPA appears to confer benefits for depression and DHA doesn't, and why the benefit is diminished at high doses, isn't terribly well understood.

It's not a simple matter of indiscriminately upping your fish oil intake. The idea that omega-3s might compete among themselves has received little attention. It looks increasingly likely that for a therapeutic effect in depression, you should be backing EPA over DHA.

> **i** While existing pharmacological treatments for depression are reasonably effective, they are not without limitations and side effects. Combining antidepressant drug therapy with EPA may significantly enhance efficacy, while reducing side effects[11, 21].

Unfortunately, most of the studies in this field have been small, and there can be no doubt that we need more in the way of large-scale, well-conducted trials. But bearing in mind the appalling rates of depression we now experience across all walks of society, we think any measures that can safely lower this burden should be promoted. And when all's said and done, there's a compelling case for us all to be regularly including oily fish in our diets and bumping up our omega-3 intakes in a bid to bolster our mental wellbeing and put a dent in the soaring depression rates. As for those suffering with depression, there is a persuasive case for including a supplement of 1g per day of EPA as part of a comprehensive treatment approach.

> **i** Depression is strongly linked with other chronic illnesses such as cardiovascular disease, diabetes, immunological abnormalities, multiple sclerosis, cancer and osteoporosis[22]. Increasing intake of oily fish/fish oils could also be beneficial in reducing many of these health problems.

Crime and nourishment

If the dearth of omega-3 fats in our modern diet could be affecting our mood, is it possible that it could be affecting our behaviour, too? In an experiment with Capuchin monkeys, when their dietary omega-3 availability was reduced, they were observed to develop severe behavioural disturbances, violence and self-inflicted injury[23]. Okay, we're not monkeys, but it does raise some questions. It's all too easy to just assume that our diets are completely separate from, and unrelated to, our behaviour. After all, suggesting what we eat can affect such abstract things as our thoughts, emotions, behaviours and actions appears to be bizarre. Yet the incontrovertible truth is that good nutrition is essential for many aspects of brain function[24]. Which leads us to ask a pretty outlandish question: could there be a nutritional component to aggressive and anti-social behaviour?

And the answer looks to be a big yes. Those countries with the highest intake of seafood have the lowest levels of homicide[25]. A high dietary intake of DHA and consumption of oily fish have been associated with a lower likelihood of hostility in young adults[26]. In substance abusers EPA (2.25g per day) and DHA (500mg per day) for three months produced significant decreases in anger and anxiety levels[27]. Giving EPA (1g per day) to women with borderline personality disorder reduced their aggression and severity of depression[28].

You start to get the picture, which leads us on to two intriguing studies that have ignited interest in how our intake of nutrients can modify behaviour. A study of 231 prisoners at a young offenders institute in Aylesbury in the UK, found that administering nutritional supplements – providing broadly the daily needs of vitamins and minerals, along with essential fatty acids – resulted in a 26% reduction in offences compared to those not receiving the supplements[29]. Indeed, those prisoners who took the nutritional supplements for at least two weeks committed 37% fewer serious offences (e.g. violence).

These findings have been replicated in a second rigorous study involving 221 young adult offenders incarcerated in eight Dutch prisons. Daily supplementation with a combination of vitamins and minerals (a standard multivitamin, similar to the UK study) and fatty acids (including 400mg of both EPA and DHA) for 30–90 days was investigated. Despite the prisoners not perceiving any change in their behaviour, there was a 34% reduction in reported incidents in those receiving the supplements, compared with a 14% increase in the control group[30].

Now prison food might not have the best reputation, but the fact is that many criminals are likely to have a better dietary status during imprisonment than they do out on the streets, especially for those prisoners.with a drug and/or alcohol addiction[30]. We can only wonder what the implications are for anti-social behaviour among swathes of society with our modern-day diets deficient in omega-3 fats and other key micronutrients. With tongue only slightly in cheek, perhaps it's high time we revolutionized the whole business of custodial sentencing by bringing in a plea of 'not guilty by reason of malnourishment, Your Honour'. Maybe it would act as the catalyst for the integration of nutrition-based strategies for both the prevention of criminal behaviour and a more enlightened rehabilitation of offenders.

> **i** Some, although not all, children with symptoms of ADHD (attention deficit hyperactivity disorder) are likely to benefit from omega-3 supplementation, and EPA, rather than DHA, is likely to be most effective in such cases[31].

Oiling the brain

For most people, the spectre of dementia in later life is simply terrifying. The fact that it is a disease process spanning many years, indeed decades, has got researchers interested in whether its initiation and progression could be lessened through diet. And what food do you think is right up there at the top of the list? Of course, we're talking fish, and most notably its rich concentration of the omega-3 fat DHA. With ageing, and especially among patients with Alzheimer's disease, DHA levels in the brain tend to decrease[32], which opens up the suggestion that a drop in DHA might contribute to the slowdown in memory and other cognitive functions with age.

> **i** Established wisdom has it that the decline in our cognitive faculties doesn't begin until old age, with no cognitive decline before the age of 60. However, a recent study of British civil servants shows that it is already evident in middle age, starting from the age of 45, and possibly even earlier[33]. Once again, this illustrates how important it is to start prevention early by following a healthy diet and lifestyle.

The results of numerous epidemiological studies support this theory[34]. Famously, a prospective study from a geographically defined community in Chicago reported that subjects who consumed fish once per week or more had 60% less risk of Alzheimer's disease compared with those who rarely or never ate fish[35]. Accompanying these findings are results from the Hordaland Health Study, a large population-based study of elderly people in Western Norway, which showed that consumers of fish had better cognitive function than non-consumers, and furthermore that this was strongly dose-dependent, with the maximum effect observed at an intake of approximately 75g of fish per day[36].

So how might fish be working its magic? There are lots of fancy 'mechanisms' to explain just how omega-3 fish oils, most notably DHA, reduce the risk of dementia. Topping the list are their anti-inflammatory effects (noting that chronic inflammation is a hallmark of Alzheimer's disease)[37]. Additionally, DHA inhibits the production, accumulation and toxicity of amyloid ß, the characteristic 'plaque' that builds up in the brain in Alzheimer's disease[38]. DHA is also thought to interfere with tau kinases and tau pathology, which are regarded as integral aspects of the neurodegenerative process[34]. We could go on...

There's just one snag, and this is that intervention trials of fish oils in patients with Alzheimer's disease have largely been ineffective. This is obviously disappointing, but perhaps not so surprising. Once again, we have to delve a bit deeper into the research to really understand what's going on here.

DHA is vital for brain development in early growth and the degree of uptake has been linked to visual development, social skills, motor skills and cognitive functioning. It's very likely that it is in youth, even childhood, that we reach what we could call our 'peak brain development'; thereafter the developmental 'window' is closed and all we can do then is try to slow the decline in our mental functioning as we age. This might be by a healthy diet and lifestyle, including, as we've just seen, a regular intake of fish rich in omega-3 fats. But when Alzheimer's disease is established, it may simply be too late. It's a case of closing the stable door after the horse has bolted.

But there are some glimmers of hope in the research. An RCT in Sweden found that while DHA supplementation in 174 elderly individuals with Alzheimer's disease produced no overall benefit after six months, when confined to those with very mild Alzheimer's, DHA was shown to arrest the decline in cognitive functioning[39]. A small-scale RCT examined fish oil supplements (EPA 1,080mg and DHA 720mg) in participants with mild to moderate Alzheimer's disease and those with much earlier mild cognitive impairment. Using the ADAS-cog test (a cognitive functioning test for Alzheimer's disease), no benefit was found from supplementation in Alzheimer patients, but those with mild cognitive impairment showed notable improvement[40]. In an RCT of 485 adults (average age 70) with mild memory problems, supplementation of 900mg per day DHA for 24 weeks resulted in participants making significantly fewer errors on a test that measured learning and memory performance compared with those who took a placebo[41].

So what about studies in healthy older people without signs of Alzheimer's disease? A well-conducted RCT of 867 cognitively healthy participants aged between 70 and 79 investigated whether a daily dose of EPA (200mg) and DHA (500mg) would slow the decline of cognitive functioning compared to olive oil[42]. Unfortunately, no answers were forthcoming because cognitive functioning did not decline in either group. The authors noted that the group receiving olive oil were actually getting enough dietary DHA already, which really only tells us what we already know. We're not necessarily talking about the need for fish oil supplements to gain benefits, as data from epidemiological studies report that as little as one meal of fish per week appears to proffer a significant protective effect[35]. Yet we only have to look at data from the UK to see that three-quarters of people don't consume any oily fish[43].

To sum all this up, let's look at a review of the evidence, which concluded that 'omega-3 fatty acids… cannot be recommended for patients who have already developed dementia' but endorsed 'fish consumption two to three times per week and/or the use of long-chain omega-3 fatty acid supplements such as DHA–EPA in elderly individuals who are looking for ways to maintain their cognitive function as they age[32].'

Of course, it would be foolish to reduce the potential benefits of fish to just its omega-3 content. After all, fish has a lot of other good things going on too that could ultimately prove to be neuro-protective, notably a rich offering of nutrients including niacin, vitamin D, vitamin B12 and selenium[44–48].

> **i** Regular fish consumption, alongside other components of a Mediterranean-style diet – rich in healthy unsaturated oils, fruit and vegetables, nuts, whole grains, other flavonoid-rich foods, and light-to-moderate intake of wine, but low in trans fats and sugar – looks like the best bet for an overall protective diet against dementia[49, 50].

With 81 million people expected to suffer with dementia by 2040[51], any lifestyle changes we can introduce to stem this mounting burden on our health are more than welcome. It doesn't require popping a ton of pills, just simply getting some fish into our diet on a regular basis.

THE PARTING SHOT

When it comes to 'brain' food, fish is quite the catch. But do we have to rely on all this fancy science to tell us what cultures around the world have known since time immemorial? All we're actually doing is catching up with something that's been embedded in religious and spiritual traditions for millennia, where fish is commonly portrayed as nirvana, a pure and sacred food associated with peace and healing[52]. Way before science came along, the antidepressant and calming properties of fish, and its rich content of omega-3 fats, seem to have been well known to our cultural and religious traditions. And it's high time we opened our eyes to this.

SUMMARY AND RECOMMENDATIONS

- Contrary to popular belief, the foods we eat can affect our mood, emotions and behaviours and, indeed, improve the way the brain functions with age.

- Patients with depression should discuss the appropriateness of including a supplement of EPA (1g per day) as part of their treatment with their medical practitioner, as it may help to improve symptoms and reduce the risk of other health problems linked to depression.

- Increasing the intake of omega-3 fish oils, alongside a broad range of essential vitamins and minerals, may also improve behavioural problems and reduce aggressive and anti-social behaviour.

- When it comes to the ageing brain, eating oily fish at least once per week helps stave off dementia and cognitive decline.

PART VII
PILL PLIGHT

'The work of the doctor will, in the future, be ever more that of an educator, and ever less that of a man who treats ailments.'

LORD HORDER, ROYAL PHYSICIAN AND CLINICIAN (1871–1955)

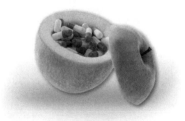

CHAPTER 18

PRESCRIPTION JUNKIES

OVERVIEW

- Rather than using drugs as a last resort, our motto has become 'drug me first, and worry about the consequences later'.

- Understand why we're a society that has become hooked on prescription drugs.

- Discover why our prescription drug culture is short-sighted and why the answers to some of our most pressing health problems can't be found in a prescription pad.

- We reveal how even preventive medicine is being hijacked by the drug industry.

- A safer, more effective and more palatable alternative exists – the best preventive medicine of all can be found in the foods we eat and the lifestyles we lead.

While I was studying pharmacy, I learned an important lesson that has stayed with me. Wide-eyed and full of enthusiasm, I eagerly got stuck into a real-life practical. Confronted with a patient suffering from acid reflux, I immediately responded with the sage advice: 'A few days of acid suppressant tablets for you sir, and if things aren't better come back to see me'. This triumphant foray into the world of dispensing drugs was short-lived, courtesy of my esteemed lecturer. Acid reflux may be a common-or-garden complaint, she patiently counselled, but investigating its cause and offering lifestyle advice to prevent it was still important. 'Remember,' she said, 'medicines are there to be used as a last resort'.

The truth is there's no such thing as a perfectly safe medicine and every drug is capable of causing side effects. Sure, some have been around a long time and we have a pretty exhaustive knowledge of them. But as for the newer ones, the full profile of adverse effects cannot be confidently known until they've spent years on the market. We're afraid to say that makes us the guinea pigs. Just take the decade 1998–2008, when 40 drugs were withdrawn from the market due to the severe side effects they caused[1]. Side effects that simply hadn't surfaced during the clinical trials designed to test their safety. Liver and heart problems accounted for 62% of the drugs withdrawn.

I could be pretty confident that those acid suppressant tablets would do the job with no untoward effects, but I now know that's not really the point. It's the false sense of security it can create, that's the problem. Fine, go ahead, take the pills, job done. What if it happens again? Don't worry, you know the tablets will take care of it. And so our trust in pharmaceutical solutions becomes embedded. With this attitude firmly entrenched, the patient need not fear future conditions. As long as there's a pill for it, all is well in the world. It might start with something reasonably trivial, like a bit of troublesome heartburn. But what if next time it's a more serious, chronic condition? A condition requiring long-term drug treatment that carries with it a higher risk of adverse side effects? Never fear, for we have another tablet that will take care of that... and as for those troublesome side effects, well, we have just the thing for those too. And so begins the slippery slope of deteriorating health and pharmaceutical dependence.

What if there was a different way? What if sometimes, all that's needed in the first place is the implementation of some carefully considered diet and lifestyle changes? Don't get us wrong, in the arsenal of patient care, drugs are vital and effective weapons, and we'd be a whole lot worse off without them. But with their risk of collateral damage, any good strategist can see that they should be the final resort. What an important lesson I learned – a worthy imperative that I figured was the backbone of patient care.

Boy was I in for a shock on entering the world of pharmacy...

Drug dependence

The inconvenient truth is that we live in a drug-dependent society. In 2008, over $234 billion was spent on prescription medications in the USA, more than double that of 1999[2]. Within the last month, 48% of Americans will have taken a prescription medication. This includes one in five children and a staggering nine in ten people aged over 60. In 1994, 2.2 million people experienced serious side effects, and more than 100,000 people died from prescription medicines, just in hospitals alone[3]. Prescription drugs are one of the biggest killers in the USA, yet, instead of serving a stark warning for prescribing practices, the consumption of prescription medicines has since increased dramatically. The stats aren't pretty and we find it more than a little difficult to reconcile this with the idea that we live in a healthy society in the twenty-first century.

Let's be clear on one thing: we're not on some all-out anti-drug crusade. There's no question of the value of medicines and that the vast majority are legitimately prescribed. In fact, there are probably many patients out there who aren't on optimal therapy and would be better served by added medications, or higher doses. But as a society, we're living in the midst of a delusion. We baulk at the dangers of recreational drugs and regard them with nothing short of horror. But we're content to remain oblivious to the harm they do once they come courtesy of a prescription pad. Instead of showing the proper respect for these potential killers, we turn to them on a whim. A culture of using drugs as a last resort has morphed into a disturbing culture of 'drug me first' prescription junkies.

It's hardly a surprise that we're popping pharmaceuticals as if they were candy. The 'drug me first' doctrine was epitomized in 1997, when the FDA (US Food and Drug Administration) allowed direct-to-consumer advertising of prescription medicines. What an absolutely astonishing decision from an organization that is 'responsible for protecting the public health' when it comes to medicine! (Thankfully, for now, this decision is unique to the USA and New Zealand; the EU and other countries still have sense enough to prohibit it.) Sure, we're all for patients taking an active interest in their health, knowing their options and being better informed. But are we really expected to believe that the best way this information is disseminated is from the people whose job it is to make profits from selling us the drugs in the first place?

With shareholders, profit margins and market share to contend with, do we really think 'big pharma' is immune to the shameless manipulation that commercial companies utilize so adeptly in ruthlessly pushing their sales?

> **i** Considering that one of the greatest public advertising expenditures by the pharmaceutical industry is for erectile dysfunction pills (not exactly the greatest health plight in the USA), you'll forgive us for thinking the industry's motives are more commercial than ethical[4].

The revolution will be televised

Advertising companies want you, the consumer, to use their products, and they'll try every last trick in the book, including playing on your emotions, to make it happen[5]. Lest we forget, in the words of Canadian economist Stephen Leacock, advertising is 'the science of arresting the human intelligence long enough to get money from it'.

For example, in the USA there is a frequently run commercial for an antidepressant (we won't name the drug but if you live in the USA and watch TV, it's run so often that you'll likely know the one we mean). It is introduced by a soporific, melancholic tune. The image: the face of a woman gazing forlornly down the camera lens. A wind-up doll becomes the analogy; its hunched, strained movements merely enduring until the encroaching, spluttering end. This is a bleak and desolate world. But after drug intervention, everything changes. The music picks up in pace and timbre. The doll moves proudly, and with purpose. A sparkle fills the woman's eyes. Sunshine and euphoria now replace the void. Oh, and a voice comes on, listing the possible side effects, which seem quite serious, and I'm pretty sure death is mentioned, but he speaks so quickly and the transformation is so overwhelming that the words seem arbitrary, irritating even. For at this time, all was good with life, and for a fleeting moment even we craved this 'wonder drug'.

There's a reason why the pharmaceutical industry spent over $4.7billion on direct-to-consumer advertising in 2008[4] (a 260% increase from 1997[6]), and there's a reason why the majority of this goes on broadcast rather than print media. This is not down to bad business sense or the sudden development of a Mother Teresa persona. It comes down to dimes and dollars, and the more people they get taking their medicines, the more money they make.

> **i** A survey found that 71% of doctors believe that direct-to-consumer advertising pressures them into prescribing drugs that they normally would not[7].

Weight loss in a pill

Let's take a prime example of how the pharmaceutical industry plays on people's emotions, and offers short-sighted pharmaceutical answers, by looking at weight loss pills. As we exposed in Part III, dieting just doesn't work long-term. Dispirited by past failures and desperate for an answer (this is where big pharma's marketing strategy really pays off), we discover there's a prescription pill that will do the job. It has been approved by the drug agencies, and prescribed by a doctor, so surely it has to be effective and safe? Well, not exactly.

Until recently, there were three main weight-loss drugs available to physicians: Acomplia® (rimonabant), Reductil® (sibutramine) and Xenical® (orlistat). Acomplia and Reductil were similar. Acting on the brain to increase satiety, they made it easier to implement a low-calorie diet, meaning patients ate less. It seems these drugs had the advantage of counteracting the adaptive thermogenesis effect seen with weight-loss diets alone, as the initial weight loss in the first six to 12 months was pretty much maintained at two years. How cool is that? Just take the pill, get back on to your favourite diet, and shedding those extra kilos is easy. Except there's one tiny hitch.

Rimonabant caused 'serious neuropsychiatric effects', with 'depressed mood disorders and anxiety' reported, along with 'increased risk of suicide during treatment'[8, 9]. Oh yeah, and rimonabant (unlike old-fashioned exercise) produced no improvement in cardiovascular outcome[9]. Rimonabant was withdrawn in November 2008, after spending two and half years on the European market. (Credit where credit is due, we must congratulate the FDA at least for not approving rimonabant for the US market in the first place.)

It wasn't long (January 2010) before sibutramine was withdrawn from the European market too, this time for actually increasing cardiovascular disease (so much for the heart-healthy benefits of weight loss). In certain patients, it caused blood-pressure spikes as high as 20mmHg and heart-rate increases of 20bpm, resulting in 16%

higher fatal or non-fatal cardiovascular complications (heart attacks and strokes)[10]. The credit the FDA gained for not approving rimonabant was negated, as they sat back for another ten months before requesting a 'voluntary' withdrawal from the manufacturer. But hey, let's not fret too much; after all, it had only been on the market for almost 13 years, with millions of prescriptions written by US physicians.

So now there is just one approved weight-loss drug on the market, but it's really nothing to boast about. Endorsed by health authorities for the obese or high-risk overweight, and touted as a long-term weight-loss solution, Xenical® (orlistat) is nothing more than the ultimate fad diet in pill form. It works by inhibiting the enzymes in the gut that break down fat, meaning that 30% of the fat eaten doesn't get absorbed.

A four-year trial of Xenical® with a low-calorie diet showed a weight loss of 5.8kg in patients who were obese[11]. On average, that is just shy of a 1.5kg weight loss per year. Okay, so it's not amazing, but maintain that for ten years and you've lost 15kg. But wait, a low-calorie diet (800kcals per day) with the added effect of inhibiting fat absorption – that's just a double whammy of reducing calories. The problem is, this drug doesn't counteract the effects of adaptive thermogenesis like rimonabant and sibutramine. Let's take a step back and have another look at this study. In the first year, patients lost a truly impressive 10.6kg, but from years two to four they gained 4.8kg . The fact that they 'only' had a 45% weight regain was most likely due to the addition of 10km walking each week[11].

In 2007, Orlistat got approved for over-the-counter sale in the USA, as the brand Alli® (half the dose of the prescription form), and was then approved in Europe in 2009. It is targeted at the overweight and obese masses (BMI >28) and promised 'for every two pounds you lose Alli® will help you lose one more'. It might sound good, but we're just back with the same old problems that beset fad diets. But this time, it just creates an even bigger calorie deficit and from one year onwards, predictably enough, the weight starts going back on.

Oh, and did we forget to mention the side effects? Excuse our oversight. Take a guess at what happens to all the malabsorbed fat? Common side effects include 'oily spotting, flatus with discharge, faecal urgency, fatty oily stool, oily evacuation, flatulence and soft stools, abdominal pain, faecal incontinence, liquid stools and increased defecation'[12]. Enough said. The gut upset can be so bad that it's thought to cause anxiety in up to 10% of people[12]. On top of that, absorption of the fat-soluble vitamins (A, D, E and K) might be impaired, and so too the healthful omega-3 fats, already in woefully short supply in our modern diets. Now we're on a roll, I guess we should quickly mention the new warning added by the FDA in 2010, that in rare cases it may cause 'severe liver injury'[13].

Perhaps of most concern when it comes to the whole obesity drug fiasco, and a prime example of how overreliant we are on drugs, is the following quote taken from a 2010 article in the prestigious *British Medical Journal (BMJ)*, written by Garth Williams, a UK Professor of Medicine:

> *Perhaps the time has come for us to face reality and admit defeat. Like climate change, nuclear waste, and other side effects of our current version of civilization, we shall just have to learn to live with obesity and its hazards*[10].

With all due respect to the esteemed professor, perhaps the time has come for us to realize that there is no quick fix and no magic bullets, and that our trust and overreliance on medications is severely and inappropriately misplaced.

Prevention in a pill

Pushing obesity to one side, we could take just about any of our major chronic diseases, say, heart disease, cancer or osteoporosis. While the diagnosis might come as a terrible shock, they didn't just happen overnight. Rather, the condition would have been brewing for years, probably decades, before finally manifesting as a heart attack, a tumour or a fracture. When the diagnosis is finally made, what we're faced with is the end product of years of progressive dysfunction in the complex machinery of the human body. When things have gone this far, how realistic is it to think that a pill will solve all of it? More often than not, the best the drugs can do is help manage the condition, buy us some time, or stop it from getting any worse. Rarely do they proffer a cure. It might not be sexy, but it's for this very reason prevention makes for such a powerful medicine.

This leads us on to the 'ingenious' idea of the polypill. In 2003, Professors Wald and Law, of London's Wolfson Institute of Preventive Medicine, suggested a blanket treatment for everyone over 55 for cardiovascular disease, based on the premise that the overwhelming majority of cardiovascular disease occurs in this age group[14]. An 'all-in-one', the polypill would be a low-dose cocktail of five different cardiovascular drugs (three for blood pressure, a statin and aspirin) and a vitamin (folic acid). The concoction was selected to modify four different cardiovascular risk factors simultaneously – blood pressure, cholesterol, blood clotting and homocysteine. It didn't matter whether you had a problem with any of these risks factors or not, this would be preventive medicine for the masses. The authors estimated that cardiovascular disease could be cut by more than 80% (although 8–15% of the population would likely suffer side effects).

In December 2004, a series of US experts gathered in Atlanta to discuss the merits of the polypill[15]. The recommendation was that clinical trials begin in the USA and Europe without further ado. The committee expressed 'excitement' at this concept of 'delivering health care in a wholly new way', especially as 'changing lifestyle is hard to achieve in current social and political environments'.

So that's it then? Changing lifestyles is all a bit too much like hard work. Let's just medicate great swathes of society instead. Once the polypill 'cures' cardiovascular disease, we'll have cancer as the new number-one killer in the world. Maybe there could be a low-dose chemotherapy polypill for that, too? Then there's diabetes, osteoporosis, Alzheimer's and arthritis, all of which urgently need to be tackled. If we could just squeeze enough drugs into a big enough pill we could stop the lot of them.

Is this really what preventive medicine has come to? A pharmaceutical pick 'n' mix? Maybe we're just naïve, but we have a very different vision of preventive medicine.

We can't help but wonder what effects a polypill that proffers 'immunity' to heart disease will have on people's behaviour? Let's face it, if we were exempt from speeding tickets when driving, there are quite a few people who would probably drive faster. Yet the accident risk is still there, and would only increase. Is the concept of the polypill really so different to that? Who cares about quitting smoking, cutting down on alcohol, starting some exercise or eating less junk if you've got a polypill to protect you? You might not get heart disease, which is great; instead you'll be hurtling for a head-on collision with any number of other chronic disease states instead.

Professors Wald and Law may have concluded that 'No other preventive method would have so great an impact on public health in the Western world', but we've got a different take on health. We already have just about the most amazing 'polypill' you could imagine. It helps prevent all prevalent Western diseases, and its key ingredients are a good diet and exercise.

Prevention on a plate

Some 18 months after Wald and Law proposed the polypill, the *British Medical Journal* published 'The Polymeal', a more natural and safer diet-based strategy[16]. The idea was to construct a diet that included a 'recipe' of cardio-protective foods that would reduce cardiovascular disease by more than 75% (putting it effectively on a par with the polypill). It sounds tasty too, consisting of dark chocolate (100g per day), fruit and vegetables (400g per day), wine (150ml per day), fish (114g four times per week), garlic (2.7g per day) and almonds (68g per day). The authors quip that 'redundant cardiologists could be retrained as Polymeal chefs and wine advisers', and while that may be a bit of light-hearted banter, there is an important underlying principle here. With a bit of ingenuity, the benefits of a wonder cure for cardiovascular disease could just as easily be replicated through food as by pharmaceuticals. As the authors so aptly put it, 'finding happiness in a frugal, active lifestyle can spare us a future of pills and hypochondria'.

Despite all of this, plans for the polypill push ahead. The results of the first world study of a polypill were published early in 2011[17]. The pill, reduced to four drugs (aspirin for platelets, lisinopril and hydrochlorothiazide for blood pressure, and simvastatin for cholesterol), was found to reduce blood pressure by 9.9/5.3mm Hg and LDL cholesterol by 20%. With the added anti-platelet effects of aspirin, this is expected to reduce the risk of coronary heart disease and stroke by 60% and 62% respectively. However, there was a big trade-off. The trial only lasted 12 weeks yet one in six patients experienced side effects, and one in 20 people had to stop the drug as the adverse events were intolerable.

It's not as though we don't have well-researched dietary alternatives either. In patients with a similar baseline blood pressure, a well-conducted RCT (the DASH study) showed that a diet high in fruit, vegetables, poultry, fish, wholegrains, nuts and low-fat dairy products – and low in red meat, sugar, saturated and total fat intake, and limited in salt – reduced blood pressure by a similar extent (8.9/4.5mm Hg)[18]. When cholesterol levels were measured it was found that LDL cholesterol levels dropped 9%[19].

Of course, as good as the DASH diet is, you needn't stop there. As you're about to see in the next chapter, greater cardio-protection could be achieved by adding plant phytostanols (2g per day) to reduce LDL levels by 10%, and eating oily fish, which proffer anti-platelet effects as well as lowering triglycerides, another important cardiovascular risk factor. Add to this the benefits of other healthy lifestyle factors – such as exercise, weight loss and smoking cessation – and it is clear to see how a comprehensive dietary and lifestyle strategy trumps the polypill big time.

Unlike the drugs, the side effects of dietary changes are all positive. Adhering closely to the DASH diet is associated with a 20% lower risk of colorectal cancer[20], and a 70% lower risk of type 2 diabetes in Caucasians[21], and as more research is published, we are expecting benefits for osteoporosis prevention to be revealed too[22].

THE PARTING SHOT

The distinction between preventive medicine and medicating society is becoming increasingly blurred. In a society defined by convenience, maybe just popping a pill is the fitting answer, irrespective of the consequences. There's a multi-billion dollar drug industry that'd be very happy with that result. But is it really such an attractive solution? Or, as we fear, is it set to unhinge the health of our society?

Since time immemorial, we've had to rely on the complex array of natural compounds found in the food we eat for real health. This won't be changing anytime soon. These, not the drugs, should be pushed to the forefront of a truly preventive system of healthcare.

SUMMARY AND RECOMMENDATIONS

- Prescription drugs have their place, but think of them more as a last resort than a first port of call.

- This is especially the case when it comes to health problems that are related to diet and lifestyle – addressing the true cause is better than popping a pill.

- Changing eating habits and behaviour is tough, but you get all the rewards without the common side effects of drugs.

- When it comes to prevention, the natural compounds found in food can take on the might of the prescription agents and usually come out on top with aplomb.

CHAPTER 19
COALITION FORCES

OVERVIEW

- Instead of being opposing forces, it's high time nutrients and drugs teamed up to maximize the benefits for patients.

- We show you how, by taking this joined-up approach, you can get the most from your medication, and at the same time, minimize adverse side effects.

- From aspirin and statins to proton pump inhibitors, we focus on the most commonly prescribed drugs and give you the lowdown on how to safely combine them with nutrients for maximum benefit.

- We also sound a note of caution when it comes to choosing your nutritional supplements – not all are created equal.

A century ago, Thomas Edison envisioned the future of medicine. In this brave new world, doctors would have no need to prescribe drugs. Instead, educating their patients about diet and lifestyle would be all that was needed to prevent disease.

Naturally, we dig Edison's vibe. It would be easy enough to take up his mantle and make this our mantra. But deep down we know that's neither realistic nor desirable. As we've seen, the way in which medicine increasingly creeps into every nook and cranny of our lives is disturbing. As too is the fact that many of our diseases could be more effectively prevented and treated by changing diet and lifestyle, not pharmaceuticals. We're backing all that to the max. Yet we prefer to live in the real world and fully accept that drugs have an important place. When used appropriately, they have an indispensable role to play in our battle against disease.

Joined-up healthcare

It's when changes to diet and lifestyle just aren't going to cut it that a drug-based approach becomes more appropriate, and sometimes pills are the best solution. Actually, we think there's an unhelpful segregation between nutrition and drugs, accompanied by the erroneous idea that you either opt for one or the other. We see it all the time. At one extreme there are people who go all out down the 'natural' route and shun drugs (sometimes with grave consequences); at the other, there are those people with prescription in hand who think there's no longer any point in following a healthy diet and lifestyle.

But the two aren't mutually exclusive. Isn't the purpose of the medical profession supposed to be the improvement of health and wellbeing? Yet how often do we hear that doctors are unwilling to embrace a holistic approach with their patients, burying their heads firmly in the sand when it comes to any talk of nutrition? Sadly, this stance is based on pure ignorance. One of the big problems with some drugs is that they deplete the body of nutrients, causing unpleasant side effects. In this scenario, all that needs to happen is that the depleted nutrients be replaced. Hardly rocket science, but how often does it happen in practice? A more 'joined-up' approach makes a whole lot more sense. Nutrition should sit there, side by side, with drug treatments. This would improve the outcome for you, the patient, would often mean that a lower dose of a drug could be used, and to top it off, help reduce unwanted side effects.

In fact, it is high time things changed, so we're going to give you the lowdown on some of the most commonly prescribed drugs. So if you want to know how to get the most benefit out of your medication, with the least adverse effects, read on.

> **i** Let's face it, with over 120 million prescriptions for aspirin, statins and proton-pump inhibitors dispensed in England alone each year[1], and hundreds of millions in the USA[2], understanding how to optimize these medicines makes sense.

Aspirin

Aspirin is a household name. It has anti-platelet effects, which basically means it prevents blood clots from forming. In patients at risk, it helps to protect against stroke and heart attack. Only low doses need to be taken to achieve this effect ($\geq$75mg), which means it's generally deemed pretty safe. However, there are still problems attributable to its use, which you'd be well advised to know about and take some simple steps to prevent.

Top of the list of problems is that aspirin can cause ulcers and bleeding, especially in the stomach. This happens even with the 'baby' doses used for cardio-protection. Low-dose aspirin therapy is implicated in 9% of cases of bleeding ulcers in people over 60[3]. What's worrying is the fact that when it comes to stomach bleeds and ulcers, you could have them but wouldn't even notice until they get progressively worse. With millions of folk popping aspirin on a daily basis, stomach bleeds are a worrying side effect. If there was a really simple, safe and affordable way to reduce that risk, you'd want to know about it, right?

Well, we know just the thing. The lining of the stomach is the body's largest store of vitamin C. Incredibly, it holds 25 times the levels found in the plasma[4]. As we said earlier, both too many and too few antioxidants are bad for you. Not only can aspirin deplete levels of vitamin C in the body, it also causes oxidative stress by increasing the free radical nitric oxide in the stomach. Simply adding in some vitamin C can restore nitric oxide back to normal levels and activates protective gut proteins[5, 6], which combines to reduce the risk of damaging your stomach lining[7, 8]. A modest supplemental dose of 100–200mg per day should confer benefits.

The other problem is that for some people, aspirin simply doesn't work. In 5–6% of people who need the drug (some scientists believe it is as high as 26%) there is no therapeutic benefit[9, 10]. This is known as 'aspirin resistance' and susceptible patients experience a near fourfold increase in cardiovascular events[11, 12]. Doctors will typically overcome this glitch by increasing the dose. But this is not always successful and means that the risk of toxicity is increased too. Upping the dose to 150mg increases the bleeding risk by over 40% and when you go higher still (300mg per day) it rises to 70%[3]. However, keeping the aspirin dose low (75mg) and adding a daily dose of fish oils (a combined dose of EPA/DHA of 2.4g per day) has been shown to achieve the same effect as increasing the aspirin dose to 325mg per day[9].

> **i** It has been suggested that fish oils thin the blood and taking them alongside aspirin increases the risk of bleeding. A comprehensive review of the studies concluded that no risk at all existed using doses of omega-3 in the range of 1–4g per day[13].

The incidence of cardiovascular disease is higher in diabetics, making them particularly strong candidates for aspirin therapy. Unfortunately, if you're diabetic, you're also more likely to be aspirin resistant. If that double whammy isn't bad enough, you're also far more likely to suffer bleeding events (by as much as 55%)[14]. That makes higher doses of aspirin pretty much a no-no. In fact, even low-dose aspirin should be used with caution by diabetics. It appears to be a no-win situation. Adding fish oils to the low-dose aspirin could enable diabetics to reap the benefit and reduce the high risk of side effects.

> **i** Concerns have been raised that fish oils reduce glucose tolerance, specifically in diabetics. A meta-analysis of 26 trials of type II diabetic patients showed no negative impact on glucose measures at up to 3g EPA/DHA per day[15].

Statins

In medicine, statins are seen as wonder drugs, no less than a modern-day panacea in cardiovascular health. Held in the highest esteem, they are the most widely prescribed cholesterol-lowering drugs. And they're effective. They drastically lower LDL cholesterol, reducing coronary events and decreasing mortality rates. Unfortunately, their use is hampered by their sizable side-effect profile. Clinical trials have found that less than 5% of people report muscle-related adverse effects, cognitive and memory problems or elevated liver enzymes[16], yet when this is translated into clinical practice, where the user characteristics are not so neatly defined and controlled, it appears that as many as 20% experience adverse effects[16]. When you consider that one in four adults over 45 now take a statin (a tenfold increase over 14 years)[17], these side effects quickly become a substantial public health problem. Needless to say, as the dose increases, so does the toxicity, which makes it desirable to prescribe the lowest possible dose to patients.

With the side effects of statins firmly in our mind, we can't help but be confused that recommendations for plant stanols (part of the phytosterol group) are not more prevalent. These occur naturally in plants and are produced commercially and added to foods. You've probably seen cholesterol-lowering spread or yogurts advertised on TV, and that's all we're talking about, nothing fancier. It just so happens that plant stanols are the perfect complement to statin therapy, but how often do you hear doctors recommending them to their patients? If it would mean taking a lower dose of statins, you'd think they'd jump at the chance.

> **i** The evidence for phytosterols is so strong that the EU has authorized health claims to be made for them as a functional food, an approval it doesn't give out too easily.

Whereas statins work on the liver to reduce cholesterol production, the plant stanols prevent cholesterol being absorbed in the gut. Combining a plant stanol with a statin creates the perfect one–two knockout strategy for high cholesterol levels. For a patient already on statins, taking a product that contains 2–2.5g of plant stanols daily reduces LDL cholesterol by a further 10% or more[18, 19]. Compare these results with the effects of doubling the dose of a statin drug, which would typically only bring about a further 6–7% drop in LDL cholesterol[20, 21]. It gets better. Unlike the statins, plant stanols are virtually free of any side effects. Even if you're not on statins but have high cholesterol (say, over 5mmol/L or 200mg/dl), incorporating plant stanol-containing products into your diet will bring benefits[22, 23].

Plant stanols have been shown to have small effects on lowering body levels of the beneficial carotenoids (primarily beta carotene)[24, 25]. This can easily be overcome by consuming a diet rich in fruit and vegetables, of which at least one serving has a high carotenoid content (e.g. carrots, sweet potatoes, pumpkins, tomatoes, apricots, kale, spinach or broccoli).

> **i** Some companies use plant sterols instead of stanols in their products. The cholesterol-lowering effects are initially the same, but there is a suggestion that sterols may contribute to the furring-up of arteries and actually promote coronary heart disease[26–28], as well as becoming less effective at lowering cholesterol over time[18, 29]. We therefore recommend that you only purchase products containing 'stanols'.

i Make sure that you don't take more than 2–2.5g of plant stanols a day. Increased intake exerts no extra benefit but will cost you more money. It has been shown to be extremely difficult to ingest this amount on a daily basis through spreads[30], requiring multiple servings per day, and thus we recommend consumption through yoghurt drinks containing the recommended 2g per serving.

The problem with statins, and indeed much of what we hear about coronary heart disease today, focuses on LDL cholesterol as the only baddie. The fact is that all cholesterol, with the exception of HDL, is harmful when high. Ideally, what we should really be talking about is 'non-HDL cholesterol' – that's your total cholesterol minus your 'good' HDL cholesterol. This includes LDL cholesterol, and also VLDL cholesterol.

The thing about VLDL cholesterol is that it carries triglycerides, an established cardiovascular risk factor. So, what you find is that, for every 1% reduction in non-HDL cholesterol from taking cholesterol-lowering drugs, there's a 1% decrease in the risk of coronary heart disease[31]. But the problem with statins is that while they can reduce VLDL/triglyceride levels, their effects are not overly strong and often require high doses, which as we know is undesirable. The upshot is that while you may have achieved ideal LDL levels on your statin therapy, your risk of heart disease can still be high[32]. Data from the USA shows that about one third of the population has triglyceride levels above 150mg/dl and 16% above 200mg/dl, which is classified as high risk[33].

i The American Heart Association classes fasting triglyceride levels of <100mg/dl as optimal, <150mg/dl as normal and 150–200mg/dl as borderline high.

Yet again, when the pharmaceuticals fall short, we find effective remedies in food. Fish oils are already recommended by the American Heart Association (AHA) for people with coronary heart disease, with just under 1g per day of EPA/DHA reducing non-fatal heart attacks, non-fatal strokes and death by 15%[34]. The Japanese diet typically provides such an amount[35], and they have extremely low levels of coronary death. Just compare this with the average Western diet, which contains a measly 100–200mg of EPA/DHA per day[36] and where heart disease is rampant. Yet at even higher doses, fish oils are effective triglyceride-lowering agents. The AHA recommends 2–4g of EPA/DHA to be taken daily (under a doctor's supervision) to lower elevated triglycerides[33]. At the upper end of the dose range, reductions in triglycerides by as much as 30% can be expected[33]. Even the lower heart-protective doses of fish oils will still confer some, albeit attenuated, triglyceride-lowering effect[37]. Used alongside statins, the reduction in VLDL results in a much greater cardio-protective effect, negating the need for ever-increasing doses of statins.

Fish oils are safe and effective and they have now been approved as prescription drugs (for example Omacor®/Lovaza®). Why it is such a rarity for doctors to prescribe them remains a mystery. In the UK, less than half a million prescriptions are dispensed annually, compared with 50 million prescriptions for statins. So if you've got high cholesterol levels, make sure your triglycerides get measured too. If they're high, speak to your doctor about prescribing fish oils.

Something fishy going on

Asking your doctor to prescribe fish oils – what's that all about? Why not just cut out the middle man and buy them over the counter yourself? It might sound a whole lot simpler but it isn't always the smart choice. First, your doctor needs to know about the supplements you take in order to properly prescribe your medications. But there's more to it than that. All the best scientific trials – showing a triglyceride-lowering effect from fish oils – have been conducted with pharmaceutical-grade products. They use fish oil in the ethyl ester form, which provides a much higher EPA/DHA concentration (84%) compared to standard over-the-counter preparations (usually only 30%). Although all concentrations lower triglycerides, it's thought that we need the higher-concentration products for the best effects.

Then we get down to purity. Dietary supplements don't undergo the same rigorous quality analysis as prescription medicines, which go through a process of meticulous testing, and abide by strict limits for potential contaminants. Environmental nasties like heavy metals, PCBs and dioxins (all carcinogenic above certain levels) are among the potential toxins prevalent in fish oil. Needless to say, you want to avoid them if you possibly can.

While we revel in getting stuck into the 'evil' drug industry, we take great comfort in thinking that the manufacturers of our nutritional supplements are part of an altruistic cottage industry that holds our health in the highest regard. Sorry to disappoint. Studies of common brands of fish oil supplements have found huge noncompliance with recommended dioxin levels. And we really should point out that these were for mainstream sale in the UK and Ireland, not some dubious backstreet products: 12 out of 33, and ten out of 15 supplements tested were found to have levels above those deemed tolerable daily intakes[38].

In 2002 and 2006, the EU introduced new limits of exposure to these noxious contaminants. But even against the might of the EU, it seems the unscrupulous were undeterred. In 2010, a European Food Safety Authority report of more than 7,000 food and animal feed products found 8% of samples had dioxins and dioxin-like PCBs exceeding maximum EU levels, with fish-related products coming out worst of all[39]. On top of this, fish oils are very unstable. If they aren't manufactured correctly and safely, unpleasant degradation products, such as peroxides and aldehydes, can form. These not only negate the benefits of fish oils supplements, but have the potential to cause harm[40]. We're pretty sure that the last thing you'd want to be doing is taking something to prevent heart disease, only to be unwittingly increasing your chances of cancer.

Just as there are some suspect products out there, there are some top-notch, high-quality ones too, so if you are going to use over-the-counter fish oil products, don't just pick the cheapest or the first one you see. Look for the one with the highest concentration of EPA and DHA, and always check for assurances of quality – ideally the GMP (Good Manufacturing Practices) certification. This way you can be assured of the closest match to pharmaceutical standards. And remember, for a significant triglyceride-lowering effect, you need one that provides 2g plus of EPA/DHA per daily serving.

THE SCIENCE BLAST: COQ10

If you take statins, you may have seen advice to take a nutritional supplement called Coenzyme Q10 (CoQ10 for short). It's one of the few examples of healthcare professionals recommending a nutrient to complement drug therapy. CoQ10 is vital for energy (ATP) production, as well as having antioxidant properties. Statins significantly deplete serum CoQ10 levels and this has been suggested as a reason for the muscle and liver problems, fatigue and possibly even the lack of benefit in heart failure. In fact, in 1989 the pharmaceutical giant Merck filed two US patents for combining CoQ10 with statins to prevent the associated muscle and liver damage. But these patents were never acted upon.

However, studies have not shown clear benefits of giving CoQ10 alongside statins. First, and contrary to what you'll hear most people saying, statins don't actually deplete serum CoQ10 levels. CoQ10 gets carried around in LDL particles. Since statins reduce LDL levels, this will have the effect of reducing the total amount of CoQ10, too. The amount of CoQ10 per LDL particle – which is what's important – actually remains the same or even increases[41–44]. There's another glitch. Serum measurements of CoQ10 are pretty much useless. That's because levels in the serum don't correlate with intracellular levels and the effects on tissues such as the muscles or liver[41, 42, 45], the very places where statins might cause a problem. So you can begin to see why measuring serum levels and then jumping to a whole lot of conclusions is a waste of time.

Studies that have taken biopsies of muscles have shown that some depletion in cellular energy production can occur from high-dose statins, but overall studies have been rather hit and miss[41, 46, 47]. This brings us nicely on to the second problem, and a flaw that permeates the scientific research, and that's a case of bad planning. All these trials have been conducted with small populations, often less than 50, and sometimes as few as 20 subjects. But the occurrence rate for muscle problems in clinical trials is less than 5%. In science there is a useful 'rule of three', that to be 95% sure that CoQ10 depletion does not occur in the 1–5% of individuals with muscle problems we would need to test a minimum population of 60–300 plus individuals. Performing studies with fewer people simply adds up to a big fat waste of time. The truth is that we may as well take the money, go to Vegas and hit the roulette tables – red it depletes levels, black it doesn't.

Even if statins do deplete tissue levels of CoQ10, being observational findings these are just associations and still don't prove that this is what is actually causing the problems. For proof, we need to see whether adding CoQ10 cures the problem. While such 'intervention' studies have been small and poorly conducted, their findings do suggest a positive effect of CoQ10 supplementation at 100mg per day in patients with muscle-related symptoms[48, 49].

The whole field of statins and CoQ10 has woven itself into a labyrinth of confusion. However, as we disentangle fact from fiction, it does appear that, in susceptible individuals, tissue levels of CoQ10 can become depleted. While still unproven, there is a notable absence of side effects from taking CoQ10, and supplementation of 100mg per day is a prudent measure, especially for those on high-dose statins. Until more conclusive studies are published, however, a more favourable approach is to incorporate plant stanols and fish oils into your regime, which will help you to use the lowest possible dose of statins.

In Japan and certain European countries, CoQ10 has now been granted a prescriptive licence in the treatment of heart failure and ischaemic heart disease[50].

Proton Pump Inhibitors

Proton Pump Inhibitors (PPIs) shut down acid production in the stomach, making them a mainstay prescription for the treatment of ulcers and acid reflux disorders. They bring noticeable symptomatic relief and, being perceived as safe drugs, doctors have no problem in prescribing them. In fact, a rampant culture of over-prescribing exists. A staggering 113 million plus prescriptions in the USA[51] and 36 million plus prescriptions in England[1] are dispensed annually. Study authors have suggested that they are being inappropriately prescribed for 25–70% of patients[52]. What makes those stats even more disturbing is the fact that we now know these drugs charge a heavy premium on our health.

Most worryingly, their long-term use depletes calcium from the bones. The occurrence of hip and spine fracture goes up by about 45–60%, an effect observable within just one year of use[53]. In one study, taking PPIs for seven or more years was associated with almost doubling of risk of an osteoporosis-related fracture. The risk for hip fracture was almost five times greater![54] The risk has been described as being 'similar in size to those for other established osteoporotic-fracture risk factors, such as smoking, low body mass index and excessive alcohol intake[54].

The biggest problem is that it appears one can't alleviate the problem simply by taking extra calcium. A large study observed that the condition appeared in PPI users independent of calcium intake[55]. How the increased risk is conferred is not actually known, but it could be due to an interaction of the parathyroid gland and vitamin D levels. It's possible that by keeping vitamin D levels optimal, the risk will be reduced, but for now this remains unproven.

On top of this, in a small proportion of patients PPI use can deplete levels of magnesium, a mineral that is also essential for bone health[56–60]. Magnesium depletion is becoming increasingly prevalent, to the extent that the FDA now recommends testing levels before and during prolonged PPI treatment. We can only conclude that it would make a lot of sense for anyone on long-term PPI treatment to ensure a plentiful dietary supply of magnesium from foods such as green leafy vegetables, nuts, wholegrain cereals and fish.

A further problem with acid suppressant tablets is the risk of vitamin B12 deficiency. We need stomach acid to liberate B12 from our food so that we can absorb it. Studies have shown that deficiency can occur in elderly people taking PPIs[61–63], and even taking a standard dose supplement providing the daily requirement of B12 is insufficient to restore levels[63]. When it comes to PPIs, the greater the dose and the greater the duration of treatment, the greater the risk of B12 deficiency becomes.

The thing with vitamin B12 is that we don't actually need a full-blown clinical deficiency to experience adverse effects. Even moderate depletion can raise levels of homocysteine in the blood. In one study, clinical B12 deficiency occurred in about one in 10 PPI users, yet raised homocysteine levels were found in approximately one third[64]. High homocysteine levels are associated with an increased risk of a plethora of afflictions, including dementia, reduced bone density and cardiovascular disease. Long-term PPI users should have their B12 and homocysteine levels monitored. If low B12 levels are evident, oral supplementation of a dose greater than the RDA (about 4–5mcg) should be taken.

It's not just nutrient depletion that you need to be concerned about with PPI use either. Stomach acid is a pivotal defence mechanism against infection. Without acid, 'bad' pathogenic bacteria can colonize our intestine, causing infection. Clostridium Difficile is a serious infection, and its incidence is growing rapidly. It can extend hospital stays by as much as 36 days[65] and for some it can be deadly. In PPI users its occurrence is increased 74%[66]. Probiotics – such as lactobacillus acidophilus, lactobacillus casei and Sacharomyces boulardii – will colonize the gut, protecting gut integrity, as well as having antimicrobial properties that can help to reduce infection risk[67–69]. However, the effects of probiotics are short-lived – usually just one to two days – so you would need to take them for the whole period that you are using the acid-suppression therapy. Probiotics may not be suitable for some patient groups (e.g. immuno-compromised), making it important to discuss this recommendation with your physician.

THE PARTING SHOT

While drugs have an important role to play, an attitude of 'in drugs we stand alone' surely has no credible place in healthcare fit for the twenty-first century. Often they cause significant nutrient depletion, or interfere with the body's important physiological functions. More often than not, careful use of nutrients in conjunction with conventional treatments would lessen the need for high-dose drug treatments and banish many of the side effects.

It's pretty clear that, when it comes to 'total' patient care, it's high time that most doctors went back to school.

SUMMARY AND RECOMMENDATIONS

- If you take aspirin to reduce the risk of stroke and heart attack, a simple low-dose vitamin C supplement of 100–200mg per day may reduce the risk of stomach ulcers and bleeding.

- If you are among the minority of people who don't respond to low-dose aspirin, you can enhance the treatment by taking a high-dose fish oil supplement, rather than increasing the dose of aspirin, which runs the risk of unwanted side effects.

- If you have high cholesterol levels, you should consider the use of plant stanols, which are widely available in cholesterol-lowering yoghurts. These can enhance the effects of statins, which means a lower dose of medication can be used.

- If you have elevated triglycerides, a risk factor for heart disease, ask your doctor to prescribe fish oils to lower them. Prescription fish oils are preferable to over-the-counter versions, some of which are of questionable potency and purity.

- If you take high-dose statins, you may consider supplementing 100mg per day of CoQ10, although we recommend using plant stanols and fish oils first to see if they can reduce the need for high-dose statins in the first place.

- If you take PPIs, it is advisable to ensure a plentiful dietary intake of nutrients needed for bone health, including calcium and magnesium, while optimizing your vitamin D status (see Chapter 7).

- Vitamin B12 and homocysteine levels should be monitored if you take PPIs long-term – you may need a vitamin B12 supplement of 4–5mcg per day.

- If you take PPIs, you may also consider supplementing with a good-quality probiotic to keep 'bad' bacteria at bay.

- **But remember**: *all* changes affecting your medicines must first be discussed with your physician or health professional.

TWENTY-FIRST CENTURY HEALTH

'Life is really simple, but we insist on making it complicated.'

CONFUCIUS, PHILOSOPHER (551–479BC)

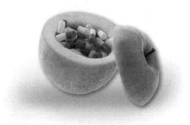

CONCLUSION

So, here we are, at the end of our journey through the diet, health and pharmaceutical industries, and all their shortcomings. There's a recurring theme throughout and that is our incessant need to overcomplicate and interfere with our health. Our message is a simple one: you cannot beat Mother Nature. By deviating away from this most basic of principles, all we end up doing is making things worse for ourselves, much worse. All the 'miracle' technological advances of recent decades may have saved us precious time and labour in our day-to-day lives, but have they provided us with a shortcut to high-level health? Who are we kidding? Such a belief is the biggest delusion of them all. Neither the fad diets, nor the pills and potions, can save us now.

The pharmaceutical, diet, food and nutritional supplement industries have all played their part in propagating this message, to the detriment of our health. We rely heavily on drugs to cure our ills, with little thought given to their side effects, or perhaps more importantly, that the origins of our health problems lie somewhere else altogether. Ultimately, the true answer to our most pressing health problems won't be found at the bottom of a pot of pills.

We've been fooled into believing that dieting can transcend our fundamental need to be active, only to backfire and fuel the obesity epidemic. We naively think we can improve on nature by bottling antioxidants and other 'super' nutrients that will rid us of our ailments and keep us forever young, when instead they only contribute to the rising rate of chronic disease. So distrustful are we of nature, that we shun the sun, only to spawn a new wave of chronic health problems in the process. So 'smart' have we become we believed we could manipulate nature to work on our terms and our terms alone, the ultimate irony being the more we meddle, the worse things get.

Take our modern diets as a prime example. We refine and process our foods until there is not a scrap of goodness left in them and then we add toxic additives in the name of flavour and preservation. So nutritionally empty have these foods become that the manufacturers have to add in colourings to stop them looking like the squalid fodder they really are. And yet, amidst this sea of junk, somehow what we end up worrying about is scaremongering the likes of meat, dairy and saturated fats – foods that have been part of our diet for millennia. It seems we don't even know what 'natural' means anymore.

Right here, right now in the twenty-first century, we've managed to confuse the most precious of things – health. We've been horribly deceived into thinking that we've evolved as a healthy society when, in fact, the opposite is true. We might be living longer, but we're not living healthier. The burden of obesity and chronic disease threatens to bring healthcare systems to their knees across the globe. We can't go on as we are. It's unsustainable in every way. Yet the reality is that the blueprint for health has already been discovered and it is available to all of us right here, right now. Sure, there will be plenty more fad diets, pharmaceutical 'cures' and nutritional 'wonder' supplements to come, but don't be fooled by them. Do we really believe that any of them will stem the tide of obesity and chronic disease we see all around us? It's only when we strip away these delusions one by one that we can begin to see them for what they are.

A PRESCRIPTION FOR HEALTH

Instead, what we're giving you is a guide for lifelong health. It's not complicated, it's really simple. It's the way things were intended. It involves getting back to basics. It's about getting back in balance with a diet in which plant and animal foods combine to provide the full spectrum of health-enhancing nutrients we need. In the few cases where our modern diet may come up short, then we recommend specific nutritional supplements, but only in the quantities that nature intended. And of course, it's not just about nourishing the body correctly, but using the body for what it was designed for – being active.

Take all these things, put them together and you have something very powerful indeed. No drug comes even close to so profoundly influencing your health and susceptibility to disease. What we're talking about is a 'prescription' that keeps your arteries healthy, fends off cancer, keeps your bones strong, combats obesity and diabetes, curbs dementia, reduces inflammation, enhances fertility, makes you happier, promotes healthy and active ageing, creates healthy children and lessens the need for pharmaceutical drugs.

What we're offering is something more sophisticated and more potent than any drug. This truly preventive medicine fit for the twenty-first century is here, on a plate, for you, your family and future generations.

THE TWENTY-FIRST CENTURY GUIDE TO EXCEPTIONAL HEALTH

1. Keep plants number one

In Essence

Wholegrains, legumes, fruit and vegetables, nuts and seeds should make up the majority of your diet for their vital, health-boosting phytonutrients.

Take Action

- Ditch the antioxidant supplements. They will never match a plant-packed diet, and they may be putting your health in jeopardy.
- Eat a rainbow of colours to ensure that you benefit from the full array of phytonutrients naturally available in fruit and vegetables.
- Making some simple dietary swaps – such as black tea for green tea and milk chocolate for dark chocolate – will boost your intake of health-enhancing flavonoids.
- Keep your grains whole and unprocessed. Restrict your refined carbohydrate intake – the white, the beige and the baked foods – as much as possible.

2. Put animal products back on the menu

In Essence

Animal products offer a source of essential nutrients not easily obtained from plant foods alone. Evidence indicates that a moderate, balanced consumption does not lead to disease.

Take Action

- There's no need to strike red meat off the menu, but limit your intake to a maximum of two servings (maximum 500g cooked weight) a week. Cook red meats at low temperatures, use marinades and dairy products, and eat a variety of flavonoid-rich plants with your meat dish.

- Avoid barbecued and charred meats.

- Processed meats – such as ham, bacon, salami, sausages and hot dogs – are a no-no. Your intake should be minimal and preferably none at all.

- Eat fish twice a week, including one serving of oily fish, for a sufficient intake of essential EPA and DHA, which are important for the body and mind alike.

- Moderate consumption of low-fat dairy products, up to three servings per day, is not linked to adverse health effects and is likely to offer protection against colon cancer.

3. Stay selenium sufficient

In Essence

Selenium is essential for health, boosting the immune system and protecting against cancer.

Take Action

- The US diet is selenium sufficient, with typically no need for supplementation.

- People living in the UK and other selenium-deficient European countries should take a daily selenium supplement – women 50–60mcg and men 100mcg – ideally in the form of selenium yeast.

4. Boost your vitamin D level

In Essence

Vitamin D is the sunshine nutrient and most of us fall short of it, putting us at unnecessary increased risk of bone disease and, very likely, cancer, immune diseases, heart disease and diabetes.

Take Action

- Smart sun exposure will keep vitamin D levels topped up in the summer.
- For the Northern American states a daily supplement of 800–1,000IU is recommended throughout the winter months.
- For the UK, Northern Europe and Canada a daily supplement of 1,100–1,200IU is recommended throughout the winter months.

5. Get active

In Essence

Humans evolved as an active species, and our recent shift to a more sedentary lifestyle is to the detriment of our waistlines and wellbeing.

Take Action

- Restricting your calories is a futile effort if you want to lose weight. Fad diets don't work. Your only option is to get active or get fatter.
- For a multitude of health benefits, aim to achieve a minimum of moderate physical activity for 30 minutes five times per week, and muscle strength training exercises twice a week.
- To lose weight, the duration and/or intensity of your exercise needs to be upped – by up to twofold – to burn sufficient calories.
- Talk to your health professional before undertaking any exercise regime.

6. Ensure the health of future generations

In Essence

The best start in life begins with good nutrition during preconception and in the womb. A healthy start can set the stage for lifelong good health and resistance to disease.

Take Action

- As you start to 'eat for two', nutritional requirements jump up. Even with a healthy diet mums-to-be need to supplement additional essential nutrients.

- The vital nutrients to get right are folic acid, iodine, selenium, vitamin D, DHA and iron – ensuring you get neither too much nor too little is the key.

- For maximum benefit, get prepared – adequate intakes of nutrients such as iodine and folic acid should be ensured before trying to conceive.

- Many of these nutrients remain essential for breastfeeding mums and in addition, breastfed babies should be given a vitamin D supplement from birth.

7. It is not medicine or nutrition

In Essence

Drugs often cause ill-effects through nutrient depletion. Harnessing the power of nutrients can mean less reliance on medicines. A holistic approach to medicine is the best prescription available.

Take Action

- Integrating nutritional strategies into standard treatment offers an effective and safe approach to treating many health problems.

- Discuss any nutrients that may complement your current healthcare regime with your physician or healthcare provider.

REFERENCES

For a full listing of unabridged references and abstracts, as well as discussion and the latest up-to-date research on all the topics covered in the book, visit us at **www.thehealthdelusion.com**

INTRODUCTION

1. Sloan, A.E. NIH State-of-the-Science Conference on Multivitamin/Mineral Supplements and Chronic Disease Prevention, 2006
2. Gahche, J. Bailey *et al. NCHS Data Brief,* 2011; (61): 1–8

CHAPTER 1: SCIENCE FICTION

1. Kurosu, H. *et al. Science,* 2005; 309(5742): 1829–33
2. Lee, S.J. *et al. Proc Natl Acad Sci USA,* 2005; 102(50): 18117–22
3. Heber-Katz, E. *et al. Philos Trans R Soc Lond B Biol Sci.,* 2004; 359(1445): 785–93
4. Bedelbaeva, K. *et al. Proc Natl Acad Sci USA.,* 2010; 107(13): 5845–50
5. Kola, I. & Landis, J. *Nat Rev Drug Discov.,* 2004; 3(8): 711–5
6. Anand, P. *et al. Mol Pharm.,* 2007; 4(6): 807–18
7. Siwak, D.R. *et al. Cancer,* 2005; 104(4): 879–90
8. O'Sullivan-Coyne, G. *et al. Br J Cancer,* 2009;101(9): 1585–95
9. Aggarwal, B.B. *et al. Clin Cancer Res.,* 2005; 11(20): 7490–8
10. Tayyem, R.F. *et al. Nutr Cancer,* 2006; 55(2): 126–31
11. Burgos-Moron, E. *et al. Int J Cancer,* 2010; 126(7): 1771–5
12. *Am J Public Health Nations Health,* 1931; 21(5): 543–5

PART I: ANTIOXIDANT ALLURE

CHAPTER 2: FOOL'S GOLD

1. Dauchet, L. *et al. J Nutr.,* 2006; 136(10): 2588–93
2. Dauchet, L. *et al. Neurology,* 2005; 65(8): 1193–7
3. Block, G. *et al. Nutr Cancer,* 1992; 18(1): 1–29.
4. Kromhout, D. *Am J Clin Nutr.,* 1987; 45 (5 Suppl): 1361–7

5. Ziegler, R.G. *J Nutr.*, 1989; 119(1): 116–22
6. Gey, K.F. *Biofactors,* 1998; 7(1–2): 113–74
7. Kardinaal, A.F. *et al. Lancet,* 1993; 342(8884): 1379–84
8. Rimm, E.B. *et al. N Engl J Med.,* 1993; 328(20): 1450–6
9. Stampfer, M.J. *et al. N Engl J Med.,* 1993; 328(20): 1444–9
10. Knekt, P. *et al. Am J Clin Nutr.,* 2004; 80(6): 1508–20
11. Myint, P.K. *et al. Am J Clin Nutr.,* 2008; 87(1): 64–9
12. Block, G. *Am J Clin Nutr.,* 1991; 53(1 Suppl): 270S–82S
13. Peto, R. *et al. Nature,* 1981; 290(5803): 201–8
14. Sloan, A.E. NIH State-of-the-Science Conference on Multivitamin/Mineral Supplements and Chronic Disease Prevention 2006
15. Gahche, J. *et al. NCHS Data Brief,* 2011; (61): 1–8
16. *Nutrition Business Journal*, 2011
17. Agriculture and Agri-Food Canada. Health and Wellness Trends for Canada and the World, 2011
18. The Alpha-Tocopherol, Beta Carotene Cancer Prevention Study Group. *N Engl J Med.,* 1994; 330(15): 1029–35
19. Gaziano, J.M. *et al. JAMA,* 2009; 301(1): 52–62
20. Sesso, H.D. *et al. JAMA,* 2008; 300(18): 2123–33
21. Waters, D.D. *et al. JAMA,* 2002; 288(19): 2432–40
22. Eidelman, R.S. *et al. Arch Intern Med.,* 2004; 164(14): 1552–6
23. Alkhenizan, A. & Hafez, K. *Ann Saudi Med.,* 2007; 27(6): 409–14
24. Lippman, S.M. *et al. JAMA,* 2009; 301(1): 39–51
25. Klein, E.A. *et al. JAMA,* 2011; 306(14): 1549–1556
26. Miller, E.R. *et al. Ann Intern Med.,* 2005; 142(1): 37–46
27. Myung, S.K. *et al. Ann Oncol.,* 2010; 21(1): 166–79
28. Bjelakovic, G. *et al. Lancet,* 2004; 364(9441): 1219–28
29. Bjelakovic, G. *et al. JAMA,* 2007; 297(8): 842–57
30. Seifried, H.E. *et al. J Nutr.,* 2004; 134(11): 3143S–63S
31. Valko, M. *et al. Chem Biol Interact.,* 2006: 160(1): 1–40
32. Gomez-Cabrera, M.C. *et al. Free Radic Biol Med.,* 2008; 44(2): 126–31
33. Ristow, M. *et al. Proc Natl Acad Sci.,* 2009; 106(21): 8665–70
34. Jiang, Q. *et al. Am J Clin Nutr.,* 2001; 74(6): 714–22
35. Helzlsouer, K.J. *et al. J Natl Cancer Inst.,* 2000; 92(24): 2018–23
36. Huang, H.Y. & Appel, L.J. *J Nutr.,* 2003; 133(10): 3137–40
37. Ye, Z. & Song, H. *Eur J Cardiovasc Prev Rehabil.,* 2008; 15(1): 26–34
38. Zhang, S. *et al. J Natl Cancer Inst.,* 1999; 91(6): 547–56
39. Levine, M. *et al. JAMA,* 1999; 281(15): 1415–23
40. Olson, J.A. & Hodges, R.E. *Am J Clin Nutr.,* 1987; 45(4): 693–703

CHAPTER 3: PLANT PROTECTION

1. Etminan, M. *et al. Cancer Epidemiol Biomarkers Prev.,* 2004; 13(3): 340–5
2. Giovannucci, E. *et al. J Natl Cancer Inst.,* 2002; 94(5): 391–8
3. Chen, L. *et al. J Natl Cancer Inst.,* 2001; 93(24): 1872–9

4. Mordente, A. *et al. Curr Med Chem.*, 2011; 18(8): 1146–63
5. Mackinnon, E.S. *et al. Osteoporosis Int.*, 2011; 22(4): 1091–101
6. Rizwan, M. *et al. Br J Dermatol.*, 2011; 164(1): 154–62
7. Freeman, V.L. *et al. Am J Epidemiol.*, 2000;151(2): 109–18
8. Lindshield, B.L. *et al. Arch Biochem Biophys.*, 2007; 458(2): 136–40
9. Seddon, J.M. *et al. JAMA*, 1994; 272(18): 1413–20
10. Ma, L. *et al. Br J Nutr.*, 2012; 107(3): 350–9
11. Chasan-Taber, L. *et al. Am J Clin Nutr.*, 1999; 70(4): 509–16
12. Brown, L. *et al.* Am J Clin Nutr., 1999; 70(4):517–24
13. Richer, S. *et al. Optometry*, 2004; 75(4): 216–30
14. Trieschmann, M. *et al. Exp Eye Res.*, 2007; 84(4): 718–28
15. Figures from nutritiondata.self.com
16. Bayard, V. *et al. Int J Med Sci.*, 2007; 4(1): 53–8
17. Miller, K.B. *et al. J Agric Food Chem.*, 2008; 56(18): 8527–33
18. Grassi, D. *et al. Am J Clin Nutr.*, 2005; 81(3): 611–4
19. Grassi, D. *et al. Hypertension*, 2005; 46(2): 398–405
20. Engler, M.B. *et al. J Am Coll Nutr.*, 2004; 23(3): 197–204
21. Desch, S. *et al. Am J Hypertens.*, 2010; 23(1): 97–103
22. Buijsse, B. *et al. Arch Intern Med.*, 2006; 166(4): 411–7
23. Janszky, I. *et al. J Intern Med.*, 2009; 266(3): 248–57
24. Egan, B.M. *et al. Hypertension*, 2010; 55(6): 1289–95
25. Hollenberg, N.K. & Fisher, N.D. *Circulation*, 2007; 116(21): 2360–2
26 Lambert, J.D. & Yang, C.S. *J Nutr.*, 2003; 133(10): 3262S–7S
27 Peters, C.M. *et al. Food Res Int.*, 2010; 43(1): 95–102
28. Sumpio, B.E. *et al. J Am Coll Surg.*, 2006; 202(5): 813–25
29. Kuriyama, S. *et al. JAMA*, 2006; 296(10): 1255–65
30. Zheng, X.X. *et al. Am J Clin Nutr.*, 2011; 94(2): 601–10
31. Wang, Z.M. *et al. Am J Clin Nutr.*, 2011; 93(3): 506–15
32. USDA Database for the Flavonoid Content of Selected Foods. 2007:http://www.
nal.usda.gov/fnic/foodcomp/Data/Flav/Flav02-1.pdf
33. Yang, C.S. & Wang, H. *Mol Nutr Food Res.*, 2011; 55(6): 819–31
34. Zheng, J. *et al. Nutr Cancer.*, 2011;63(5): 663–72.
35. Kang, H. *et al. Epidemiol Health*, 2010; 32: e2010001
36. Tang, N. *et al. Lung Cancer*, 2009; 65(3): 274–83
37. Ogunleye, A.A. *et al. Breast Cancer Res Treat.*, 2010; 119(2): 477–84
38. Dai, Q. *et al. Ann Epidemiol.*, 2010; 20(1): 74–81
39. Bettuzzi, S. *et al. Cancer Res.*, 2006; 66(2): 1234–40
40. Tsao, A.S. *et al. Cancer Prev Res* (Phila)., 2009; 2(11): 931–41
41. Wu, M. *et al. Int J Cancer*, 2009; 124(8): 1907–13
42. Sun, J. *et al. J AOAC Int.*, 2011; 94(2): 487–97
43. Hurrell, R.F. *et al. Br J Nutr.*, 1999; 81(4): 289–95
44. Zijp, I.M. *et al. Crit Rev Food Sci Nutr.*, 2000; 40(5): 371–98
45. Erdman, J.W. *et al. J Nutr.*, 2007; 137(3 Suppl 1): 718S–37S
46. Clarke, J.D. *et al. Cancer Lett.*, 2008; 269(2): 291–304
47. Voorrips, L.E. *et al. Am J Epidemiol.*, 2000; 152(11): 1081–92

48. Cohen, J.H. *et al. J Natl Cancer Inst.,* 2000; 92(1): 61–8
49. Kolonel, L.N. *et al. Cancer Epidemiol Biomarkers Prev.,* 2000; 9(8): 795–804
50. Fowke, J.H. *et al. Cancer Res.,* 2003; 63(14): 3980–6
51. Michaud, D.S. *et al. J Natl Cancer Inst.,* 1999; 91(7): 605–13
52. Tang, L. *et al. Cancer Epidemiol Biomarkers Prev.,* 2008; 17(4): 938–44
53. Zhao, B. *et al. Cancer Epidemiol Biomarkers Prev.,* 2001; 10(10): 1063–7
54. Yuan, J.M. *et al. Int J Cancer,* 1998; 77(2): 211–6
55. Nagle, C.M. *et al. Int J Cancer,* 2003; 106(2): 264–9
56. Traka, M. *et al. PLoS One.,* 2008; 3(7): e2568
57. Bonnesen, C. *et al. Cancer Res.,* 2001; 61(16): 6120–30
58. Zhang, Y. *et al. Free Radic Biol Med.,* 2005; 38(1): 70–7
59. Forester, S.C. & Lambert, J.D. *Mol Nutr Food Res.,* 2011; 55(6): 844–54

CHAPTER 4: SELENIUM: A MISSING PUZZLE PIECE

1. Rayman, M.P. *BMJ,* 1997; 314(7078): 387–8
2. Fairweather-Tait, S.J. *et al. Antioxid Redox Signal.,* 2011; 14(7): 1337–83
3. Rayman, M.P. *Br J Nutr.,* 2008; 100(2): 254–68
4. Ferlay, J. *et al. Eur J Cancer,* 2010; 46(4): 765–81
5. Karunasinghe, N. *et al. Cancer Epidemiol Biomarkers Prev.,* 2004; 13(3): 391–7
6. Kiremidjian-Schumacher, L. *et al. Biol Trace Elem Res.,* 2000; 73(2): 97–111
7. Broome, C.S. *et al. Am J Clin Nutr.,* 2004; 80(1): 154–62
8. Rayman, M.P. *Proc Nutr Soc.,* 2005; 64(4): 527–42
9. Duffield-Lillico, A.J. *et al. Cancer Epidemiol Biomarkers Prev.,* 2002; 11(7): 630–9
10. Duffield-Lillico, A.J. *et al. BJU Int.,* 2003; 91(7): 608–12
11. Lippman, S.M. *et al. JAMA,* 2009; 301(1): 39–51
12. Rayman, M.P. *Biochim Biophys Acta.,* 2009; 1790(11): 1533–40
13. Hurst, R. *et al. Am J Clin Nutr.,* 2010; 91(4): 923–31
14. Rayman, M.P. *Lancet,* 2000; 356(9225): 233–41
15. Laclaustra, M. *et al. Environ Health Perspect.,* 2009; 117(9): 1409–13

PART II: SUN SUPPLEMENT

CHAPTER 5: 'D'-FICIENT BONES

1. Holick, M.F. *N Engl J Med.,* 2007; 357(3): 266–81
2. Looker, A.C. *et al. NCHS Data Brief,* 2011; (59): 1–8
3. Hypponen, E. & Power, C. *Am J Clin Nutr.,* 2007; 85(3): 860–8
4. Ashwell, M. *et al. Br J Nutr.,* 2010; 104(4): 603–11
5. Lanham-New, S.A. *Proc Nutr Soc.,* 2008; 67(2): 163–76
6. Heaney, R.P. *Am J Clin Nutr.,* 2008; 88(2): 541S–4S
7. Vieth, R. *Ann Med.,* 2005; 37(4): 278–85
8. Steingrimsdottir, L. *et al. JAMA,* 2005; 294(18): 2336–41
9. Johnell, O. *et al. Osteoporos Int.,* 2007; 18(3): 333–7

10. Kaye, E.K. *J Am Dent Assoc.,* 2007; 138(5): 616–9
11. Cooper, C. *et al. J Nutr.,* 2005;135(11): 2728S–34S
12. Hollis, B.W & Wagner, C.L. *Am J Clin Nutr.,* 2004; 79(5): 717–26
13. Javaid, M.K. *et al. Lancet,* 2006; 367(9504): 36–43
14. Gordon, C.M. *et al. Arch Pediatr Adolesc Med.,* 2004; 158(6): 531–7
15. Guillemant, J. *et al. Osteoporosis Int.,* 1999; 10(3): 222–5
16. Lehtonen-Veromaa, M.K. *et al. Am J Clin Nutr.,* 2002; 76(6): 1446–53
17. Lehtonen-Veromaa, M.K. *et al. Am J Clin Nutr.,* 2003; 78(2): 351–2 (letter)
18. Frost, M. *et al. Clin Endocrinol (Oxf).,* 2010; 73(5): 573–80
19. Trivedi, D.P. *et al. BMJ,* 2003; 326(7387): 469
20. Bischoff-Ferrari, H.A. *et al. Arch Intern Med.,* 2009; 169(6): 551–61
21. Chapuy, M.C. *et al. N Engl J Med.,* 1992; 327(23): 1637–42
22. Avenell, A. *et al.* Cochrane Database Syst Rev., 2009(2): CD000227
23. DIPART Group *BMJ,* 2010; 340: b5463
24. Goldacre, M.J. *et al. BMJ,* 2002; 325(7369): 868–9
25. Bischoff-Ferrari, H.A. *Best Pract Res Clin Rheumatol.,* 2009; 23(6): 789–95
26. Wicherts, I.S. *et al. J Clin Endocrinol Metab.,* 2007; 92(6): 2058–65
27. Bischoff-Ferrari, H.A. *et al. BMJ,* 2009; 339: b3692
28. CDC. http://www.cdc.gov/homeandrecreationalsafety/falls/adultfalls.html

CHAPTER 6: 'D'-FICIENT BODY

1. http://www.pa-international.org/MEP_Questions.htm
2. Peller S. & Stephenson, C.S. *Am J Med Sci.,* 1937; (194): 326–33
3. Holick, M.F. & Chen, T.C. *Am J Clin Nutr.,* 2008; 87(4): 1080S–6S
4. Robsahm, T.E. *et al. Cancer Causes Control,* 2004; 15(2): 149–58
5. Porojnicu, A.C. *et al. Br J Cancer.,* 2005; 93(5): 571–4
6. Giovannucci, E. *et al. Arch Intern Med.,* 2008; 168(11): 1174–80
7. Joseph, A.J. *et al. Indian J Med Res.,* 2009; 130(2): 133–7
8. Luong, K. *et al. Diabetes Metab Res Rev.,* 2005; 21(4): 338–46
9. Vieira, V.M. *et al. Environ Health Perspect.,* 2010; 118(7): 957–61
10. Ascherio, A. *et al. Lancet Neurol.,* 2010; 9(6): 599–612
11. CDC. http://www.cdc.gov/nchs/fastats/lcod.htm
12. Eyre, H. *et al. Diabetes Care,* 2004; 27(7): 1812–24
13. Grant, W.B. *Dermatoendocrinol,* 2009; 1(1): 25–33
14. Grant, W.B. & Garland, C.F. *Anticancer Res.,* 2006; 26(4A): 2687–99
15. Heaney, R.P *et al. Arch Intern Med.,* 2011; 171(3): 266; author reply 7
16. Cancer Research UK. http://info.cancerresearchuk.org/cancerstats/keyfacts/Allcancerscombined
17. Freedman, D.M *et al. J Natl Cancer Inst.,* 2007; 99(21): 1594–602
18. Gorham, E.D. *et al. Am J Prev Med.,* 2007; 32(3): 210–6
19. Chen, P. *et al. Breast Cancer Res Treat.,* 2010; 121(2): 469–77
20. Yin, L. *et al. Eur J Cancer,* 2010; 46(12): 2196–205
21. CDC. www.cdc.gov
22. Manson, J.E. *et al. N Engl J Med.,* 2011; 364(15): 1385–7

23. Wactawski-Wende, J. *et al. N Engl J Med.,* 2006; 354(7): 684–96
24. Chlebowski, R.T. *et al. J Natl Cancer Inst.,* 2008; 100(22): 1581–91
25. Lappe, J.M. *et al. Am J Clin Nutr.,* 2007; 85(6): 1586–91
26. Ojha, R.P. *et al. Am J Clin Nutr.,* 2007; 86(6): 1804–5; author reply 5–6
27. Sood, M.M & Sood, A.R. *Am J Clin Nutr.,* 2007; 86(5): 1549; author reply 49–50
28. Schabas, R. *Am J Clin Nutr.,* 2008; 87(3): 792; author reply 3–4
29. Bolland, M.J. & Reid, I.R. *Am J Clin Nutr.,* 2008; 87(3): 792–3; author reply 3–4
30. CDC. http://www.cdc.gov/heartdisease/facts.htm
31. Heidenreich, P.A. *et al. Circulation,* 2011; 123(8): 933–44
32. Wang, T.J. *et al. Circulation,* 2008; 117(4): 503–11
33. Forman, J.P. *et al. Hypertension,* 2007; 49(5): 1063–9
34. Pilz, S. *et al. Stroke,* 2008; 39(9): 2611–3
35. Pilz, S. *et al. J Clin Endocrinol Metab.,* 2008; 93(10): 3927–35
36. Souberbielle, J.C. *et al. Autoimmun Rev.,* 2010; 9(11): 709–15
37. Trivedi, D.P. *et al. BMJ,* 2003; 326(7387): 469
38. Prince, R.L. *et al. Arch Intern Med.,* 2008; 168(1): 103–8
39. Palomer, X. *et al. Diabetes Obes Metab.,* 2008; 10(3): 185–97
40. Wild, S. *et al, Diabetes Care,* 2004; 27(5): 1047–53
41. CDC. http://www.cdc.gov/features/diabetesfactsheet
42. Mitri, J. *et al Eur J Clin Nutr.,* 2011; 65(9): 1005–15
43. Pittas, A.G. *et al. J Clin Endocrinol Metab.,* 2007; 92(6): 2017–29
44. Nikooyeh, B. *et al. Am J Clin Nutr.,* 2011; 93(4): 764–71
45. Dahlquist, G. & Mustonen, L. *Int J Epidemiol.,* 1994; 23(6): 1234–41
46. Moltchanova, E.V. *et al. Diabet Med.,* 2009; 26(7): 673–8
47. Littorin, B. *et al. Diabetologia,* 2006; 49(12): 2847–52
48. Zipitis, C.S. & Akobeng, A.K. *Arch Dis Child.,* 2008; 93(6): 512–7
49. Hypponen, E. *et al. Lancet,* 2001; 358(9292): 1500–3
50. Urashima, M. *et al. Am J Clin Nutr.,* 2010; 91(5): 1255–60
51. Autier, P. & Gandini, S. *Arch Intern Med.,* 2007; 167(16): 1730–7

CHAPTER 7: 'D'-LIVERED

1. Holick, M.F. *Am J Clin Nutr.,* 2004; 80(6 Suppl): 1678S–88S
2. Hanley, D.A. *et al. CMAJ,* 2010; 182(12): E610–8
3. Holick, M.F. *N Engl J Med.,* 2007; 357(3): 266–81
4. Riker, A.I. *et al. Ochsner J.,* 2010; 10(2): 56–65
5. Cancer Research UK http://info.cancerresearchuk.org/cancerstats/types/skin/riskfactors
6. CDC. Cancer Statistics. http://www.cdc.gov
7. Czarnecki, D. *et al. Clin Exp Dermatol.,* 2009; 34(5): 624–5
8. Engelsen, O. *et al. Photochem Photobiol.,* 2005; 81(6): 1287–90
9. *Rep Health Soc Subj.,* (Lond), 1991; 41: 1–210
10. Webb, A.R. *et al. J Clin Endocrinol Metab.,* 1988; 67(2): 373–8
11. International Agency for Research on Cancer Working Group on artificial ultraviolet (UV) light and skin cancer, *Int J Cancer,* 2007; 120(5): 1116–22

12. Rapuri, P.B. *et al. J Clin Endocrinol Metab.,* 2002; 87(5): 2024–32
13. Hypponen, E. & Power, C. *Am J Clin Nutr.,* 2007; 85(3): 860–8
14. Cashman, K.D. *et al. Am J Clin Nutr.,* 2008; 88(6): 1535–42
15. Looker, A.C. *et al. NCHS Data Brief,* 2011; (59): 1–8
16. USDA ERS. http://www.ers.usda.gov/publications/ldp/xlstables/pccons-P.xls
17. Cranney, A. *et al. Am J Clin Nutr.,* 2008; 88(2): 513S–9S
18. Wortsman, J. *et al. Am J Clin Nutr.,* 2000; 72(3): 690–3
19. Blum, M. *et al. J Am Coll Nutr.,* 2008; 27(2): 274–9
20. Flegal, K.M. *et al. JAMA,* 2010; 303(3): 235–41
21. Heaney, R.P. *et al. Am J Clin Nutr.,* 2003; 77(1): 204–10
22. Weber, F. *Prog Clin Biol Res.,* 1981; 77: 119–35
23. Mulligan, G.B. & Licata, A. *J Bone Miner Res.,* 2010; 25(4): 928–30
24. Binkley, N. *et al. J Clin Endocrinol Metab.,* 2007; 92(6): 2130–5
25. IOM *Dietary Reference Intakes for Calcium and Vitamin D,* Washington, DC: The National Academies Press, 2011
26. Ford, E.S. *et al. V Int J Epidemiol.,* 2011; 40(4): 998–1005
27. Melamed, M.L. *et al. Arch Intern Med.,* 2008; 168(15): 1629–37
28. Tuohimaa, P. *et al. Int J Cancer,* 2004; 108(1): 104–8
29. Helzlsouer, K.J. *Am J Epidemiol.,* 2010; 172(1): 4–9
30. Abnet, C.C. *et al. Cancer Epidemiol Biomarkers Prev.,* 2007; 16(9): 1889–93

PART III: DIET DISCREPANCIES

CHAPTER 8: FAD DIETS: A PACT WITH THE DEVIL

1. Kopelman, P. *Obes Rev.,* 2007; 8 Suppl 1: 13–7
2. Foster, G.D. *et al. N Engl J Med.,* 2003; 348(21): 2082–90.
3. Samaha, F.F. *et al. N Engl J Med.,* 2003; 348(21): 2074–81
4. Stem, L. *et al. Ann Intern Med.,* 2004; 140(10): 778–85
5. Smith, S.R. *N Engl J Med.,* 2009; 361(23): 2286–8
6. Dansinger, M.L. *et al. JAMA,* 2005; 293(1): 43–53
7. Heshka, S. *et al. JAMA,* 2003; 289(14): 1792–8
8. Rosenbaum, M. & Leibel, R.L. *Int J Obes (Lond).,* 2010; 34 Suppl 1: S47–55
9. Dulloo, A.G. *Int J Obes (Lond).,* 2007; 31(2): 201–3
10. Sacks, F.M. *et al. N Engl J Med.,* 2009; 360(9): 859–73
11. Hill, A.J. *Br J Nutr.,* 2004; 92 Suppl 1: S15–8
12. Morton, G.J. *et al. Nature,* 2006; 443(7109): 289–95
13. Rosenbaum, M. *et al. Am J Clin Nutr.,* 2008; 88(4): 906–12

CHAPTER 9: THE AGE OF THE SLOTH

1. DEFRA. 2007; http://www.defra.gov.uk/statistics/files/defra-stats-food-family-annual-200506.pdf
2. Gray-Donald, K. *et al. Can J Public Health.,* 2000; 91(5): 381–5

3.   Heini, A.F. & Weinsier, R.L. *Am J Med.,* 1997; 102(3): 259–64
4.   CDC. http://www.cdc.gov/mmwr/preview/mmwrhtml/mm5304a3.htm
5.   Racette, S.B. *et al. Obesity (Silver Spring),* 2008; 16(8): 1826–30
6.   Slyper, A.H. *J Clin Endocrinol Metab.,* 2004; 89(6): 2540–7
7.   Wu, Y. *BMJ,* 2006; 333(7564): 362–3
8.   Zhai, F. *et al. Nutr Rev.,* 2009; 67 Suppl 1: S56–61
9.   House of Commons Health Committee, 2004 http://www.publications. parliament.uk/pa/cm200304/cmselect/cmhealth/23/23.pdf
10. Martinez-Gonzalez, M.A. *et al. Int J Obes Relat Metab Disord.,* 1999; 23(11): 1192–201
11. Fang, J. *et al. Am J Prev Med.,* 2003; 25(4): 283–9
12. Kimm, S.Y. *et al. Lancet,* 2005; 366(9482): 301–7
13. Slentz, C.A. *et al. Obesity (Silver Spring),* 2009; 17 Suppl 3: S27–33
14. Haskell, W.L. *et al. Med Sci Sports Exerc.,* 2007; 39(8): 1423–34
15. Leitzmann, M.F. *et al. Arch Intern Med.,* 2007; 167(22): 2453–60
16. Blair, S.N. *et al. Am J Clin Nutr.,* 2004; 79(5): 913S–20S
17. CDC. *Growing Stronger – Strength Training for Older Adults*, 2002
18. CDC. http://www.cdc.gov/nchs/fastats/exercise.htm.
19. NHS. 2010; http://www.ic.nhs.uk/webfiles/publications/opad10/Statistics_on_ Obesity_Physical_Activity_and_Diet_England_2010.pdf
20. Troiano, R.P. *et al. Med Sci Sports Exerc.,* 2008; 40(1): 181–8
21. Rosenbaum, M. & Leibel, R.L. *Int J Obes (Lond).,* 2010; 34 Suppl 1: S47–55
22. Hollowell, R.P. *et al. Med Sci Sports Exerc.,* 2009; 41(8): 1640–4
23. Tremblay, A. *et al. Int J Obes.,* 1990; 14(1): 75–84
24. Weiss, E.P. *et al. Rejuvenation Res.,* 2008; 11(3): 605–9
25. Hunter G.R. *et al. Obesity (Silver Spring).* 2006;14(11):2018–25.
26. Pratley R. *et al. J Appl Physiol.* 1994;76(1):133–7.
27. Knab, A.M. *et al. Med Sci Sports Exerc.,* 2011; 43(9): 1643–8
28. Martins, C. *et al. Int J Obes (Lond).,* 2008; 32(9): 1337–47
29. Ross, R. *et al. Ann Intern Med.,* 2000; 133(2): 92–103
30. Donnelly, J.E. *et al. Arch Intern Med.,* 2003; 163(11): 1343–50
31. Catenacci V.A. *et al. Obesity (Silver Spring),* 2008; 16(1):153–61.
32. Catenacci, V.A. *et al. Obesity (Silver Spring),* 2011; 19(6): 1163–70
33. Sigal, R.J. *et al. Diabetes Care,* 2006; 29(6): 1433–8

CHAPTER 10: THE SKINNY ON FAT

1.   Pischon, T. *et al. N Engl J Med.,* 2008; 359(20): 2105–20
2.   Kershaw, E.E. & Flier, J.S. *J Clin Endocrinol Metab.,* 2004; 89(6): 2548–56
3.   Fox, C.S. *et al. Circulation,* 2007; 116(1): 39–48
4.   Schapira, D.V *et al. Cancer,* 1994; 74(2): 632–9
5.   Fontana, L. *et al. Diabetes,* 2007; 56(4): 1010–3
6.   Thomas, E.L. *et al. Obesity (Silver Spring),* 2012; 20(1): 76–87
7.   Personal Correspondence with Professor Jimmy Bell
8.   Porter, S.A. *et al. Diabetes Care,* 2009; 32(6): 1068–75

9. Lassek, W. & Gaulin S.J.C. *Evolution and Human Behavior,* 2008; 29: 28–36
10. Lee, D.C. *et al. Br J Sports Med.,* 2009;43(1): 49–51
11. Wildman, R.P. *et al. Arch Intern Med.,* 2008; 168(15): 1617–24
12. O'Donovan, G. *et al. Int J Obes (Lond).,* 2009; 33(12): 1356–62
13. Lee, C.D. *et al. Am J Clin Nutr.,* 1999; 69(3): 373–80
14. Sui, X. *et al. JAMA,* 2007; 298(21): 2507–16
15. Blair, S.N. & Church, T.S. *JAMA,* 2004; 292(10): 1232–4
16. Blair, S.N & Brodney, S. *Med Sci Sports Exerc.,* 1999; 31(11 Suppl): S646–62
17. Slentz, C.A. *et al. Obesity (Silver Spring),* 2009; 17 Suppl 3: S27–33

PART IV: ANIMAL ATTACKS

CHAPTER 11: WHAT'S THE MATTER WITH MILK?

1. Parkin, D.M. *et al. CA Cancer J Clin.,* 2005; 55(2): 74–108
2. Althuis, M.D. *et al. Int J Epidemiol.,* 2005; 34(2): 405–12
3. Ganmaa, D. *et al. Int J Cancer.,* 2002; 98(2): 262–7
4. Qin, L.Q. *et al. Nutr Cancer.,* 2004; 48(1): 22–7
5. Wang, Y. & Li, S. *Food Nutr Bull.,* 2008; 29(3): 172–85
6. Zhu, Y.G. *et al. Environ Sci Technol.,* 2011; 45(12): 5099–104
7. World Cancer Research Fund/American Institute for Cancer Research. *Food, Nutrition, Physical Activity, and the Prevention of Cancer: a Global Perspective*, Washington DC: AICR, 2007
8. Gao, X. *et al. J Natl Cancer Inst.,* 2005; 97(23): 1768–77
9. Allen, N.E. *et al. Br J Cancer,* 2008; 98(9): 1574–81
10. Giovannucci, E. *et al. Int J Cancer,* 2007; 121(7): 1571–8
11. Bailey, R.L. *et al. J Nutr.,* 2010; 140(4): 817–22
12. Bolland, M.J. *et al. BMJ,* 2010; 341: *c.*3691
13. Giovannucci, E. *et al. Cancer Res.,* 1998; 58(3): 442–7
14. Tseng, M. *et al. Am J Clin Nutr.,* 2005; 81(5): 1147–54
15. Baron, J.A. *et al. Cancer Epidemiol Biomarkers Prev.,* 2005; 14(3): 586–9
16. Shi, R. *et al. Br J Cancer,* 2001; 85(7): 991–6
17. Hankinson, S.E. *et al. Lancet,* 1998; 351(9113): 1393–6
18. Heaney, R.P. *et al. J Am Diet Assoc.,* 1999; 99(10): 1228–33
19. Yan, L. & Spitznagel, E.L. *Am J Clin Nutr.,* 2009; 89(4): 1155–63
20. Hilakivi-Clarke, L. *et al. J Nutr.,* 2010; 140(12): 2326S–34S
21. Khalil, D.A. *et al. J Nutr.,* 2002; 132(9): 2605–8
22. Pala, V. *et al. Am J Clin Nutr.,* 2009; 90(3): 602–12
23. Dong, J.Y. *et al. Breast Cancer Res Treat.,* 2011; 127(1): 23–31
24. Jacobson, E.A. *et al. Cancer Res.,* 1989; 49(22): 6300–3
25. Chen, P. *et al. Breast Cancer Res Treat.,* 2010; 121(2): 469–77
26. Aune, D. *et al. Ann Oncol.,* 2012; 23(1): 37–45
27. Holt, P.R. *et al. Nutr Cancer,* 2001; 41(1–2): 150–5
28. Holt, P.R. *et al. JAMA,* 1998; 280(12): 1074–9

CHAPTER 12: WHAT'S THE BEEF WITH MEAT?

1. World Cancer Research Fund/American Institute for Cancer Research. *Food, Nutrition, Physical Activity, and the Prevention of Cancer: a Global Perspective,* Washington DC: AICR, 2007
2. Alexander, D.D. *et al. Am J Clin Nutr.,* 2009; 89(5): 1402–9
3. www.cdc.gov
4. Rohrmann, S. *et al. Am J Clin Nutr.,* 2009; 89(5): 1418–24
5. Bastide, N.M. *et al. Cancer Prev Res (Phila).,* 2011; 4(2): 177–84
6. Kabat, G.C. *et al. Int J Cancer.,* 2009; 124(10): 2430–5
7. Ferrucci, L.M. *et al. Br J Cancer.,* 2009; 101(1): 178–84
8. Pala, V. *et al. Am J Clin Nutr.,* 2009; 90(3): 602–12
9. Larsson, S.C. *et al. Eur J Cancer.,* 2009; 45(17): 3042–6
10. Appleby, P.N. *et al. Int J Obes Relat Metab Disord.,* 1998; 22(5): 454–60
11. Appleby, P.N. *et al. Public Health Nutr.,* 2002; 5(5): 645–54
12. Alexander, D.D. *et al. Nutr J.,* 2010; 9: 50
13. Corpet, D.E. *Meat Sci.,* 2011; 89(3): 310–6
14. Smith, J.S. *et al. J Food Sci.,* 2008; 73(6): T100–5
15. Persson, E. *et al. Food Chem Toxicol.,* 2003; 41(11): 1587–97
16. Gibis, M.J. *Agric Food Chem.,* 2007; 55(25): 10240–7
17. Balogh, Z. *et al. Food Chem Toxicol.,* 2000; 38(5): 395–401
18. Nerurkar, P.V. *et al. Nutr Cancer.,* 1999; 34(2): 147–52
19. Melo, A. *et al. J Agric Food Chem.,* 2008; 56(22): 10625–32
20. Hallberg, L. *et al. Am J Clin Nutr.,* 1991; 53(1): 112–9
21. Ma, Q. *et al. J Nutr.,* 2010; 140(6): 1117–21

CHAPTER 13: CAN PLANT-BASED DIETS PROVIDE IT ALL?

1. Fraser, G.E. *Am J Clin Nutr.,* 2009; 89(5): 1607S–12S
2. Craig, W.J. & Mangels, A.R. *J Am Diet Assoc.,* 2009; 109(7): 1266–82
3. http://www.visualeconomics.com/food-consumption-in-america_2010-07-12 2010
4. USDA. http://www.usda.gov/factbook/chapter2.htm
5. NHS. http://www.nhs.uk/Livewell/5ADAY/Pages/Why5ADAY.aspx
6. Wynn E. *et al. Proc Nutr Soc.* 2010; 69(1):166–73
7. Kelly, J.H. Jr. & Sabate, J. *Br J Nutr.,* 2006; 96 Suppl 2: S61–7
8. Slavin, J. *Proc Nutr Soc.,* 2003; 62(1): 129–34
9. Fardet, A. *Nutr Res Rev.,* 2010; 23(1): 65–134
10. Anderson, J.W. & Major A.W. *Br J Nutr.,* 2002; 88 Suppl 3: S263–71
11. Rizkalla, S.W. *et al. Br J Nutr.,* 2002; 88 Suppl 3: S255–62
12. Mann, J. *BMJ.* 2009; 339: b2507
13. Haddad, E.H. & Tanzman, J.S. *Am J Clin Nutr.* 2003; 78(3 Suppl): 626S–32S
14. Key, T.J. *et al. BMJ,* 1996; 313(7060): 775–9
15. Gilsing, A.M. *et al. Eur J Clin Nutr.,* 2010; 64(9): 933–9
16. Key, T.J. *et al. Proc Nutr Soc.,* 2006; 65(1): 35–41

17. Herrmann, W. *et al. Clin Chem.*, 2001;47(6):1094–101
18. Craig, W.J. *Am J Clin Nutr.*, 2009; 89(5): 1627S–33S
19. Stark, A.H. *et al. Nutr Rev., 2008;* 66(6): 326–32
20. Rosell, M.S. *et al. Am J Clin Nutr.*, 2005; 82(2): 327–34
21. Kornsteiner, M. *et al. Ann Nutr Metab.*, 2008; 52(1): 37–47
22. Craig, W.J. *Nutr Clin Pract.*, 2010; 25(6): 613–20
23. Dunn-Emke, S.R. *et al. J Am Diet Assoc.*, 2005; 105(9): 1442–6
24. Outila, T.A. *et al. J Am Diet Assoc.*, 2000; 100(4): 434–41
25. Smith, A.M. *Int J Nurs Pract.*, 2006; 12(5): 302–6
26. Appleby, P. *et al. Eur J Clin Nutr.*, 2007; 61(12): 1400–6
27. Gibson, R.S. *Am J Clin Nutr.*, 1994; 59(5 Suppl): 1223S–32S
28. Larsson, C.L. & Johansson G.K. *Am J Clin Nutr.*, 2002; 76(1): 100–6
29. Letsiou, S. *et al. Eur J Nutr., 2010;* 49(8): 465–72
30. Teucher, B. *et al. Int J Vitam Nutr Res.*, 2004; 74(6): 403–19
31. Krajcovicova-Kudlackova, M. *et al. Ann Nutr Metab.*, 2003; 47(5): 183–5
32. Andersson, M. *et al. Best Pract Res Clin Endocrinol Metab.*, 2010; 24(1): 1–11
33. Lazarus, J.H. & Smyth, P.P. *Lancet,* 2008; 372(9642): 888
34. Lee, S.M. *et al. Br J Nutr.* 1994; 72(3): 435–46

PART V: GENERATION GAINS

CHAPTER 14: YOU ARE WHAT YOUR MOTHER ATE

1. Chen, A. *et al. Int J Epidemiol.*, 2006; 35(1): 121–30
2. Barker, D.J. & Osmond, C. *Lancet*, 1986; 1(8489): 1077–81
3. Barker, D. *BMJ,* 2003; 327(7429): 1428–30
4. Osmond, C. *et al. BMJ.* 1993; 307(6918): 1519–24
5. Gillman, M.W. *et al. Pediatrics,* 2003; 111(3): e221–6
6. Ehrenberg, H.M. *et al. Am J Obstet Gynecol.*, 2004; 191(3): 964–8
7. Huxley, R. *et al. Am J Clin Nutr.*, 2007; 85(5): 1244–50
8. Rasmussen, K.M. *Annu Rev Nutr.*, 2001; 21: 73–95
9. Fowden, A.L. *et al. Physiology (Bethesda),* 2006; 21: 29–37
10. Lesage, J. *et al. Endocrinology,* 2001; 142(5): 1692–702
11. Langley-Evans, S.C. *Proc Nutr Soc.*, 2001; 60(4): 505–13
12. Wells, J.C. *Biol Rev Camb Philos Soc.*, 2007; 82(1): 143–72
13. Armitage, J.A. *et al. J Physiol.*, 2004; 561(Pt 2): 355–77
14. Vaag, A. *Int J Gynaecol Obstet.*, 2009; 104 Suppl 1: S32–4
15. Ong, K.K. *et al. BMJ,* 2000; 320(7240): 967–71
16. Ong, K.K. & Loos R.J. *Acta Paediatr.*, 2006; 95(8): 904–8
17. Huxley, R.R. *et al. J Hypertens.*, 2000; 18(7): 815–31
18. Eriksson, J.G. *et al. BMJ,* 1999; 318(7181): 427–31
19. Cianfarani, S. *et al. Arch Dis Child Foetal Neonatal Ed.*, 1999; 81(1): F71–3
20. Barker, D.J. *et al. N Engl J Med.*, 2005; 353(17): 1802–9
21. Huxley, R. *et al. Lancet.* 2002; 360(9334): 659–65

22. Roseboom, T. *et al. Early Hum Dev.,* 2006; 82(8): 485–91
23. Neugebauer, R. *JAMA,* 2005; 294(5): 621–3
24. Richards, M. *et al. BMJ,* 2001; 322(7280): 199–203
25. Richards, M. *et al. Int J Epidemiol.,* 2002; 31(2): 342–8
26. Kristensen, P. *et al. Int J Epidemiol.,* 2004; 33(4): 849–56
27. Phillips, D.I. *et al. BMJ,* 2001; 322(7289): 771
28. Fall, C.H. *et al. Food Nutr Bull.,* 2009; 30(4 Suppl): S533–46
29. Christian, P. & Stewart C.P. *J Nutr.,* 2010; 140(3): 437–45
30. Rich-Edwards, J.W. *et al. BMJ,* 2005; 330(7500): 1115

CHAPTER 15: NOURISHING THE NEXT GENERATION

1. The International Council for the Control of Iodine Deficiency Disorders http://www.iccidd.org/pages/iodine-deficiency.php
2. Caldwell, K.L. *et al. Thyroid,* 2011; 21(4): 419–27
3. Henderson, L. *et al.* E. London: The Stationary Office, 2003
4. Glinoer, D. *Public Health Nutr.,* 2007; 10(12A): 1542–6
5. WHO. *Assessment of iodine deficiency disorders and monitoring their elimination. A guide for programme managers, Third Edition*, 2007
6. Lazarus, J.H. & Smyth, P.P. *Lancet,* 2008; 372(9642): 888
7. Vanderpump M.P. *et al. Lancet,* 2011; 377(9782): 2007–12
8. Delange, F. *Thyroid,* 1994; 4(1): 107–28
9. WHO. *Iodine deficiency in Europe: A continuing public health problem*, 2007
10. Kooistra, L. *et al. Pediatrics,* 2006; 117(1): 161–7
11. Zimmermann, M.B. *Endocr Rev.,* 2009; 30(4): 376–408
12. Costeira, M.J. *et al. J Pediatr.,* 2011; 159(3): 447–53
13. Pop, V.J. *et al. Clin Endocrinol (Oxf).,* 2003; 59(3): 282–8
14. Vermiglio, F. *et al. J Clin Endocrinol Metab.,* 2004; 89(12): 6054–60
15. Zimmermann, M.B. *Am J Clin Nutr.,* 2009; 89(2): 668S–72S
16. Zimmermann, M. & Delange, F. *Eur J Clin Nutr.,* 2004; 58(7): 979–84
17. Gregory, C.O. *et al. Thyroid,* 2009; 19(9): 1019–20
18. Bath, S.C. *et al. Br J Nut.,* 2011; 1–6. [Epub ahead of print]
19. Krajcovicova-Kudlackova, M. *et al. Ann Nutr Metab.,* 2003; 47(5): 183–5
20. Remer, T. *et al. Br J Nutr.,* 1999; 81(1): 45–9
21. Craig, W.J. & Mangels, A.R. *J Am Diet Assoc.,* 2009; 109(7): 1266–82
22. Lightowler, H.J. & Davies, G.J. *Br J Nutr.,* 1998; 80(6): 529–35
23. Teas, J. *et al. Thyroid,* 2004; 14(10): 836–41
24. Barrington, J.W. *et al. Br J Obstet Gynaecol.,* 1996; 103(2): 130–2
25. Kumar, K.S. *et al. J Obstet Gynaecol.,* 2002; 22(2): 181–3
26. Mistry, H.D. *et al. Am J Obstet Gynecol.,* 2012; 206(1): 21–30
27. Rayman, M.P. *et al. Am J Obstet Gynecol.,* 2003; 189(5): 1343–9
28. Rayman, M.P *et al. CMAJ.* 2011; 183(5): 549–55
29. Tara, F. *et al. J Obstet Gynaecol.,* 2010; 30(1): 30–4
30. Arthur, J.R. *et al. Nutr Res Rev.,* 1999; 12(1): 55–73
31. Bodnar, L.M. *et al. J Clin Endocrinol Metab.,* 2007; 92(9): 3517–22

32. Mannion, C.A. *et al. CMAJ.,* 2006; 174(9): 1273–7
33. Hoogenboezem, T. *et al. Pediatr Res.,* 1989; 25(6): 623–8
34. Wagner, C.L. *et al. Breastfeed Med.,* 2006; 1(2): 59–70
35. Hollis, B.W. & Wagner, C.L. *Public Health Nutr.,* 2011; 14(4): 748–9
36. Hollis, B.W. & Wagner, C.L. *Am J Clin Nutr.,* 2004; 80(6 Suppl): 1752S–8S
37. Wagner, C.L. & Greer, F.R. *Pediatrics,* 2008; 122(5): 1142–52
38. Greer, F.R. *Am J Clin Nutr.,* 2008; 88(2): 529S–33S
39. Giapros, V.I. *et al. Eur J Clin Nutr.,* 2011
40. Misra, M. *et al. Pediatrics,* 2008; 122(2): 398–417
41. Siafarikas, A. *et al. Arch Dis Child.,* 2011; 96(1): 91–5
42. Perrine, C.G. *et al. Pediatrics.,* 2010; 125(4): 627–32
43. NHS 2009. http://www.lnds.nhs.uk/Library/dh_111302.pdf
44. Taylor, J.A. *et al. Pediatrics,* 2010; 125(1): 105–11
45. Alwan, N. & Cade J. *Perspect Public Health,* 2011; 131(5): 207–8
46. Scholl, T.O. *Am J Clin Nutr.,* 2005; 81(5): 1218S–22S
47. Cogswell, M.E. *et al. Am J Clin Nutr.,* 2003; 78(4): 773–81
48. Siega-Riz, A.M. *et al. Am J Obstet Gynecol.,* 2006; 194(2): 512–9
49. CDC. http://www.cdc.gov/mmwr/preview/mmwrhtml/00051880.htm (1998)
50. Viteri, F.E. & Berger, J. *J Nutr Rev.,* 2005; 63(12 Pt 2): S65–76
51. Mei, Z. *et al. Am J Clin Nutr.,* 2011; 93(6): 1312–20
52. Bothwell, T.H. *Am J Clin Nutr.,* 2000; 72(1 Suppl): 257S–64S
53. Milman, N. *et al. Acta Obstet Gynecol Scand.,* 1999; 78(9): 749–57
54. Pena-Rosas, J.P. & Viteri F.E. *Cochrane Database Syst Rev.,* 2009; 4: CD004736
55. Weinberg, E.D. *Med Hypotheses,* 2009; 73(5): 714–5
56. Walsh, T. *et al. Clin Chem Lab Med.,* 2011; 49(7): 1225–30
57. Carlson, S.E. *Am J Clin Nutr.,* 2009; 89(2): 678S–84S
58. Makrides, M. *Prostaglandins Leukot Essent Fatty Acids.,* 2009; 81(2–3): 171–4
59. Duttaroy, A.K. *Prog Lipid Res.,* 2009; 48(1): 52–61
60. Jordan, R.G. *J Midwifery Women's Health,* 2010; 55(6): 520–8
61. Smith, K.M. & Sahyoun, N.R. *Nutr Rev.,* 2005; 63(2): 39–46
62. Hibbeln, J.R. *et al. Lancet,* 2007; 369(9561): 578–85
63. Obican, S.G. *et al. FASEB J.,* 2010; 24(11): 4167–74
64. Wolff, T. *et al. Ann Intern Med.,* 2009; 150(9): 632–9
65. CDC. http://www.cdc.gov/ncbddd/folicacid/data.html
66. Talaulikar, V. & Arulkumaran, S. *Obstetrics, Gynaecology & Reproductive Medicine,* 2011; 21(5): 147–8
67. Smith, A.D. *et al. Am J Clin Nutr.,* 2008; 87(3): 517–33

PART VI: FAILING FATS

CHAPTER 16: A BIG FAT MISTAKE

1. FDA. 2010; http://www.fda.gov/ForConsumers/ConsumerUpdates/ucm202611.htm

2. FSA. 2009; http://www.food.gov.uk/multimedia/pdfs/publicattitudestofood.pdf
3. FSA. 2009; http://www.food.gov.uk/news/pressreleases/2009/feb/launchsatfatcampaign
4. Expert Panel on Detection, Evaluation, and Treatment of High Blood Cholesterol in Adults, *JAMA,* 2001; 285(19): 2486–97
5. Appel, L.J. *et al. JAMA,* 2005; 294(19): 2455–64
6. Siri-Tarino, P.W. *et al. Curr Atheroscler Rep.,* 2010; 12(6): 384–90
7. Siri-Tarino, P.W. *et al. Am J Clin Nutr.,* 2010; 91(3): 535–46
8. Yamagishi, K. *et al. Am J Clin Nutr.,* 2010; 92(4): 759–65
9. CDC. http://www.cdc.gov/mmwr/preview/mmwrhtml/mm5304a3.htm
10. Mensink, R.P. *et al. Am J Clin Nutr.,* 2003; 77(5): 1146–55
11. Jakobsen, M.U. *et al. Am J Clin Nutr.,* 2009; 89(5): 1425–32
12. Siri-Tarino, P.W. *et al. Am J Clin Nutr.,* 2010; 91(3): 502–9
13. McBride, P. *Curr Atheroscler Rep.,* 2008; 10(5): 386–90
14. Krauss, R.M. *et al. Am J Clin Nutr.,* 2006; 83(5): 1025–31; quiz 205
15. Jakobsen, M.U. *et al. Am J Clin Nutr.,* 2010; 91(6): 1764–8
16. Ludwig, D.S. *JAMA,* 2002; 287(18): 2414–23
17. Hu, F.B. *Am J Clin Nutr.,* 2010; 91(6): 1541–2
18. Mozaffarian, D. *et al. PLoS Med.,* 2010; 7(3): e1000252
19. Harris, W.S. *et al. Circulation,* 2009; 119(6): 902–7
20. Czernichow, S. *et al. Br J Nutr.,* 2010; 104(6): 788–96
21. Expert Panel on Detection, Evaluation, and Treatment of High Blood Cholesterol in Adults, *Circulation,* 2002; 106(25): 3143–421
22. Hussein, N. *et al. J Lipid Res.,* 2005; 46(2): 269–80
23. Fritsche, K.L. *Prostaglandins Leukot Essent Fatty Acids*., 2008; 79(3–5): 173–5
24. Blasbalg, T.L. *et al. Am J Clin Nutr.,* 2011; 93(5): 950–62
25. Ramsden, C.E. *et al. Br J Nutr.,* 2010; 104(11): 1586–600
26. GISSI-Prevenzione trial, *Lancet,* 1999; 354(9177): 447–55
27. Grundy, S.M. *Circulation,* 2003; 107(14): 1834–6
28. Mozaffarian, D. *Lancet,* 2007; 369(9567): 1062–3.
29. Smith, K.M. & Sahyoun N.R. *Nutr Rev.,* 2005; 63(2): 39–46
30. Kris-Etherton, P.M. *et al. Am J Clin Nutr.,* 2000; 71(1 Suppl): 179S–88S
31. Kris-Etherton, P.M, *et al. Circulation,* 2002; 106(21): 2747–57
32. Daviglus, M.L. *et al. N Engl J Med.,* 1997; 336(15): 1046–53
33. Whelton, S.P. *et al. Am J Cardiol.,* 2004; 93(9): 1119–23
34. ISSFAL Statement. 2004; http://archive.issfal.org/index.php/lipid-matters-mainmenu-8/issfal-policy-statements-mainmenu-9/23-issfal-policy-statement-3
35. Calder, P.C. *Am J Clin Nutr.,* 2006; 83(6 Suppl): 1505S–19S
36. Chapkin, R.S. *et al. Prostaglandins Leukot Essent Fatty Acids,* 2009; 81(2–3): 187–91
37. Kremer, J.M. *Am J Clin Nutr.,* 2000; 71(1 Suppl): 349S–51S
38. Goldberg, R.J. & Katz J. *Pain,* 2007; 129(1–2): 210–23
39. Davis, B.C. & Kris-Etherton P.M. *Am J Clin Nutr.,* 2003; 78(3 Suppl): 640S–6S
40. Lopez-Miranda, J. *et al. Nutr Metab Cardiovasc Dis.,* 2010; 20(4): 284–94
41. Yashodhara, B.M. *et al. Postgrad Med J.,* 2009; 85(1000): 84–90
42. Dayton, S. *et al. Circulation,* 1965; 32(6): 911–24

43. Pischon, T. *et al. Circulation,* 2003; 108(2): 155–60
44. Munakata, M. *et al. Tohoku J Exp Med.,* 2009; 217(1): 23–8
45. Geppert, J. *et al. Lipids,* 2005; 40(8): 807–14

CHAPTER 17: BRAIN DRAIN

1.   *Nature,* 2011; 477(7363): 132
2.   CDC. http://www.cdc.gov/mentalhealthsurveillance/fact_sheet.html
3.   CDC. http://www.cdc.gov/Features/dsDepression
4.   Anderson, I.M. *J Affect Disord.,* 2000; 58(1): 19–36
5.   Bloch, M.H. & Hannestad, J. *Mol Psychiatry,* 2011; Sep 20 (epub ahead of print)
6.   Hibbeln J.R. *Lancet,* 1998; 351(9110): 1213
7.   Tanskanen, A. *et al. Psychiatr Serv.,* 2001; 52(4): 529–31
8.   Appleton, K.M. *et al. Am J Clin Nutr.,* 2006; 84(6): 1308–16
9.   Lin, P.Y. *et al. Biol Psychiatry,* 2010; 68(2): 140–7
10. Edwards, R. *et al. J Affect Disord.,* 1998; 48(2–3): 149–55
11. Nemets, B. *et al. Am J Psychiatry.,* 2002; 159(3): 477–9
12. Peet, M. & Horrobin, D.F. *Arch Gen Psychiatry.,* 2002; 59(10): 913–9
13. Nemets, H. *et al. Am J Psychiatry,* 2006; 163(6): 1098–100
14. Su, K.P. *et al. J Clin Psychiatry,* 2008; 69(4): 644–51
15. Marangell, L.B. *et al. Am J Psychiatry,* 2003; 160(5): 996–8
16. Silvers, K.M. *et al. Prostaglandins Leukot Essent Fatty Acids,* 2005; 72(3): 211–8
17. Grenyer, B.F. *et al. Prog Neuropsychopharmacol Biol Psychiatry,* 2007; 31(7): 1393–6
18. Rogers, P.J. *et al. Br J Nutr.,* 2008; 99(2): 421–31
19. Martins, J.G. *J Am Coll Nutr.,* 2009; 28(5): 525–42
20. Sublette, M.E. *et al. J Clin Psychiatry,* 2011; 72(12):1577–84
21. Jazayeri, S. *et al. Aust N Z J Psychiatry,* 2008; 42(3): 192–8
22. Horrobin, D.F. & Bennett, C.N. *Prostaglandins Leukot Essent Fatty Acids,* 1999; 60(4): 217–34
23. Fiennes, R.N. *et al. J Med Primatol.,* 1973; 2(3): 155–69
24. Gomez-Pinilla, F. *Nat Rev Neurosci.,* 2008; 9(7): 568–78
25. Hibbeln, J.R. *World Rev Nutr Diet.,* 2001; 88: 41–6
26. Iribarren, C. *et al. Eur J Clin Nutr.,* 2004; 58(1): 24–31
27. Buydens-Branchey, L. *et al. Prog Neuropsychopharmacol Biol Psychiatry*, 2008; 32(2): 568–75
28. Zanarini, M.C. & Frankenburg, F.R. *Am J Psychiatry,* 2003; 160(1): 167–9
29. Gesch, C.B. *et al. Br J Psychiatry,* 2002; 181: 22–8
30. Zaalberg, A. *et al. Aggress Behav.,* 2010; 36(2): 117–26
31. Bloch, M.H. & Qawasmi, A. *J Am Acad Child Adolesc Psychiatry,* 2011; 50(10): 991–1000
32. Fotuhi, M. *et al. Nat Clin Pract Neurol.,* 2009; 5(3): 140–52
33. Singh-Manoux, A. *et al. BMJ,* 2012; 344: d7622
34. Cole, G.M. *et al. Prostaglandins Leukot Essent Fatty Acids*, 2009; 81(2–3): 213–21
35. Morris, M.C. *et al. Arch Neurol.,* 2003; 60(7): 940–6

36. Nurk, E. *et al. Am J Clin Nutr.,* 2007; 86(5): 1470–8
37. Calder, P.C. *Am J Clin Nutr.,* 2006; 83(6 Suppl): 1505S–19S
38. Lim, G.P. *et al. J Neurosci.,* 2005; 25(12): 3032–40
39. Freund-Levi, Y. *et al. Arch Neurol.,* 2006; 63(10): 1402–8
40. Chiu, C.C. *et al. Prog Neuropsychopharmacol Biol Psychiatry,* 2008; 32(6): 1538–44
41. Yurko-Mauro, K. *et al. Alzheimer's Dement.,* 2010; 6(6): 456–64
42. Dangour, A.D. *et al. Am J Clin Nutr.,* 2010; 91(6): 1725–32
43. COT http://cot.food.gov.uk/pdfs/fishreport2004full.pdf
44. Morris, M.C. *et al. J Neurol Neurosurg Psychiatry,* 2004; 75(8): 1093–9
45. Llewellyn, D.J. *et al. Arch Intern Med.,* 2010; 170(13): 1135–41
46. Dickens, A.P. *et al. CNS Drugs.,* 2011; 25(8): 629–39
47. Vogiatzoglou, A. *et al. Neurology,* 2008; 71(11): 826–32
48. Berr, C. *et al. J Am Geriatr Soc.,* 2000; 48(10): 1285–91
49. Corsinovi, L. *et al. Mol Nutr Food Res.,* 2011; 55 Suppl 2: S161–72
50. Solfrizzi, V. *et al. Expert Rev Neurother.,* 2011; 11(5): 677–708
51. Ferri, C.P. *et al. Lancet,* 2005; 366(9503): 2112–7
52. Reis, L.C. & Hibbeln, J.R. *Prostaglandins Leukot Essent Fatty Acids.,* 2006; 75(4–5): 227–36

PART VII: PILL PLIGHT

CHAPTER 18: PRESCRIPTION JUNKIES

1. MacDonald, J.S. & Robertson, R.T. *Toxicol Sci.,* 2009; 110(1): 40–6
2. CDC. http://www.cdc.gov/nchs/data/databriefs/db42.htm
3. Lazarou, J. *et al. JAMA,* 1998; 279(15): 1200–5
4. Congressional Budget Office, 2009 http://www.cbo.gov/ftpdocs/105xx/doc10522/12-02-DrugPromo_Brief.pdf
5. Wolfe, S.M. *N Engl J Med.,* 2002; 346(7): 524–6
6. Donohue, J.M. *et al. N Engl J Med.,* 2007; 357(7): 673–81
7. Rosenthal, M.B. *et al. N Engl J Med.,* 2002; 346(7): 498–505
8. Christensen, R. *et al. Lancet;* 2007; 370(9600): 1706–13
9. Topol, E.J. *Lancet,* 2010; 376(9740): 517–23
10. Williams, G. *BMJ,* 2010; 340: c.824.
11. Torgerson, J.S. *et al. Diabetes Care,* 2004; 27(1): 155–61
12. *Evid Based Nurs.,* 2010; 13(3): 98–100
13. FDA. Questions and Answers, 2010; http://www.fda.gov/Drugs/DrugSafety/PostmarketDrugSafetyInformationforPatientsandProviders/ucm213040.htm.
14. Wald, N.J. & Law, M.R. *BMJ,* 2003; 326(7404): 1419
15. Smith, R. *BMJ,* 2005; 330(7481): 8
16. Franco, O.H. *et al. BMJ,* 2004; 329(7480): 1447–50
17. Rodgers, A. *et al. PLoS One.,* 2011; 6(5): e19857
18. Sacks, F.M. *et al. N Engl J Med.,* 2001; 344(1): 3–10

19. Obarzanek, E. *et al. Am J Clin Nutr.,* 2001; 74(1): 80–9
20. Fung, T.T. *et al. Am J Clin Nutr.,* 2010; 92(6): 1429–35
21. Liese, A.D. *et al. Diabetes Care,* 2009; 32(8): 1434–6
22. Lin, P.H. *et al. J Nutr.,* 2003; 133(10): 3130–6

CHAPTER 19: COALITION FORCES

1. The NHS Information Centre P.S.U. 2010
2. IMS Health. 2010; http://www.pharmacytimes.com/issue/pharmacy/2010/May2010/RxFocusTopDrugs-0510
3. Weil, J. *et al. BMJ,* 1995; 310(6983): 827–30
4. Schulz, H.U. *et al. Int J Clin Pharmacol Ther.,* 2004; 42(9): 481–7
5. Becker, J.C. *et al. Biochem Biophys Res Commun.,* 2003; 312(2): 507–12
6. Konturek, P.C. *et al. J Physiol Pharmacol.,* 2006; 57 Suppl 5: 125–36
7. Pohle, T. *et al. Aliment Pharmacol Ther.,* 2001; 15(5): 677–87
8. Dammann, H.G. *et al. Aliment Pharmacol Ther.,* 2004; 19(3): 367–74
9. Lev, E.I. *et al. J Am Coll Cardiol.,* 2010; 55(2): 114–21
10. Hovens, M.M. *et al. Am Heart J.,* 2007; 153(2): 175–81
11. Krasopoulos, G. *et al. BMJ,* 2008; 336(7637): 195–8
12. Snoep, J.D. *et al. Arch Intern Med.,* 2007; 167(15): 1593–9
13. Harris, W.S. *Am J Cardiol.,* 2007; 99(6A): 44C–6C
14. Baigent, C. *et al. Lancet,* 2009; 373(9678): 1849–60
15. Friedberg, C.E. *et al. Diabetes Care,* 1998; 21(4): 494–500
16. Maningat, P. & Breslow J.L. *N Engl J Med.,* 2011;365(24): 2250–1
17. CDC. *Statin drug use in the past 30 days among adults 45 years of age and over, by sex and age: USA, 1988–1994, 1999–2002 and 2005–2008*
18. de Jong, A. *et al. Br J Nutr.,* 2008; 100(5): 937–41
19. Scholle, J.M. *et al. J Am Coll Nutr.,* 2009; 28(5): 517–24
20. Blair, S.N. *et al. Am J Cardiol.,* 2000; 86(1): 46–52
21. Roberts, W.C. *Am J Cardiol.,* 1997; 80(1): 106–7
22. Expert Panel on Detection, Evaluation and Treatment of High Blood Cholesterol in Adults. *JAMA,* 2001; 285(19): 2486–97
23. Abumweis, S.S. *et al. Food Nutr Res.,* 2008; 52
24. Hallikainen, M.A. *et al. Eur J Clin Nutr.,* 2000; 54(9): 715–25
25. Hallikainen, M.A. *et al. Eur J Clin Nutr.,* 1999; 53(12): 966–9
26. Ketomaki, A. *et al. Clin Chim Acta.,* 2005; 353(1–2): 75–86
27. Sudhop, T. *et al. Metabolism,* 2002; 51(12): 1519–21
28. Rajaratnam, R.A. *et al. J Am Coll Cardiol.,* 2000; 35(5): 1185–91
29. O'Neill, F.H. *et al. Am J Cardiol.,* 2005; 96(1A): 29D–36D
30. Eussen, S.R. *et al. Public Health Nutr.,* 2011; 14(10): 1823–32
31. Robinson, J.G. *et al. J Am Coll Cardiol.,* 2009; 53(4): 316–22
32. Watts, G.F. & Karpe, F. *Heart,* 2011; 97(5): 350–6
33. Miller, M. *et al. Circulation,* 2011; 123(20): 2292–333
34. GISSI Prevenzione Trial *Lancet,* 1999; 354(9177): 447–55.
35. Mozaffarian D. *Lancet,* 2007; 369(9567):1062–3.

36. Kris-Etherton, P.M. *et al. Am J Clin Nutr.*, 2000; 71(1 Suppl): 179S–88S
37. Harris, W. *European Heart Journal Supplements,* 2001; (3): D59–D61
38. FSA. 2002; http://www.food.gov.uk/multimedia/pdfs/26diox.pdf
39. EFSA. *EFSA Journal,* 2010; 8(3): 1385
40. Rupp, H. *Adv Ther.*, 2009; 26(7): 675–90
41. Paiva, H. *et al. Clin Pharmacol Ther.*, 2005; 78(1): 60–8
42. Avis, H.J. *et al. J Pediatr.*, 2011; 158(3): 458–62.
43. Liu, C.S. *et al. Nutr Res.*, 2010; 30(2):118–24
44. Colquhoun, D.M. *et al. Eur J Clin Invest.*, 2005; 35(4): 251–8
45. Knauer, M.J. *et al. Circ Res.*, 2010; 106(2): 297–306
46. Laaksonen, R. *et al. Am J Cardiol.*, 1996; 77(10): 851–4
47. Laaksonen, R. *et al. Clin Pharmacol Ther.*, 1995; 57(1): 62–6
48. Kelly, P. *et al. J Am Coll Cardiol.*, 2005; (45): 3A
49. Caso, G. *et al. Am J Cardiol.*, 2007; 99(10): 1409–12
50. Pepe, S. *et al. Mitochondrion.*, 2007; 7 Suppl: S154–67
51. Katz, M.H. *Arch Intern Med.,* 2010; 170(9): 747–8
52. Forgacs, I. & Loganayagam, A. *BMJ,* 2008; 336(7634): 2–3
53. Vestergaard, P. *et al. Calcif Tissue Int.,* 2006; 79(2): 76–83
54. Targownik, L.E. *et al. CMAJ.,* 2008; 179(4): 319–26
55. Gray, S.L. *et al. Arch Intern Med.,* 2010; 170(9): 765–71
56. FDA Drug Safety Communication. 2011; http://www.fda.gov/Drugs/DrugSafety/ucm245011.htm
57. Wallach, S. *Magnes Trace Elem.,* 1990; 9(1): 1–14
58. Rude, R.K. & Gruber, H.E. *J Nutr Biochem.,* 2004; 15(12): 710–6
59. Sojka, J.E. & Weaver, C.M. *Nutr Rev.,* 1995; 53(3): 71–4
60. Aydin, H. *et al. Biol Trace Elem Res.,* 2010; 133(2): 136–43
61. Howden, C.W. *J Clin Gastroenterol.,* 2000; 30(1): 29–33
62. Force, R.W. *et al. Ann Pharmacother.,* 2003; 37(4): 490–3
63. Dharmarajan, T.S. *et al. J Am Med Dir Assoc.,* 2008; 9(3): 162–7
64. Hirschowitz, B.I. *et al. Aliment Pharmacol Ther.,* 2008; 27(11): 1110–21
65. McFarland, L.V. *Anaerobe,* 2009; 15(6): 274–80
66. Howell, M.D. *et al. Arch Intern Med.,* 2010; 170(9): 784–90
67. McFarland, L.V. *Am J Gastroenterol.,* 2006; 101(4): 812–22
68. Hickson, M. *et al. BMJ,* 2007; 335(7610): 80
69. Gao, X.W. *et al. Am J Gastroenterol.,* 2010; 105(7): 1636–41

INDEX

This index is in word-by-word alphabetical order.

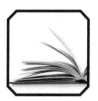

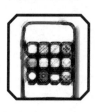

ABOUT THE AUTHORS

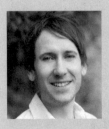

Glen Matten is a Nutritional Therapist with a Masters Degree in Nutritional Medicine from the University of Surrey, where he graduated with Distinction. Glen's firm belief in the importance of diet in promoting health and preventing disease is fundamental to his work, which spans private consultancy, teaching and lecturing, research and corporate workshops. Glen is in clinical practice in London and Norwich, where he is dedicated to improving the health of the individuals he works with through carefully tailored nutritional programmes.

Glen combines his passion for nutritional medicine with being a full-on foodie, with a fresh approach to nutrition that has led to frequent forays into the media, including numerous TV appearances. Glen is an established writer who regularly contributes to a number of publications, and is the author of *The 100 Foods You Should Be Eating*.

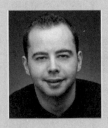

Aidan Goggins is an Irish pharmacist with a Master's Degree in Nutritional Medicine. He is a firm believer in the necessity of a holistic approach to achieve true health, and that medicine alone is insufficient to stem the rising burden of chronic disease. He is a strong advocate of complementing medicine with nutrition and lifestyle changes to improve patient outcome and reduce undesirable side effects.

It was while studying for his Masters in Nutritional Medicine that Aidan was aggrieved to discover how much compelling nutrition research was not finding its way to the public. Either being ignored, misinterpreted or simply not noticed, the end result was the same; the public was getting an extremely raw deal. Heart disease, cancer, diabetes and more – if only the right advice was being given we would be able to halt many of these fatal maladies at their inception.

www.thehealthdelusion.com
www.healthuncut.com